"Ladies and Gentlemen, this is your Surgeon speaking..."

EXPLORING THE 'HUMAN FACTOR' IN
AVIATION AND SURGERY.

GEOFF HAY

'Ladies and Gentlemen, this is your Surgeon speaking'
Exploring the Human Factor in Aviation and Surgery

First published in Australia by Geoff Hay 2019
geoffhay@supersonicperformance.com.au

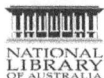

A catalogue record for this
book is available from the
National Library of Australia

ISBN: 978-0-6485154-0-1 (pbk)
ISBN: 978-0-6485154-1-8 (ebk)

Typesetting and design by Publicious Book Publishing
Published in collaboration with Publicious Book Publishing
www.publicious.com.au

Dedication

To my wonderful, enthusiastic, energetic and supportive family who constantly remind me what a great team looks like, and to my son Andrew for your computer, proof reading and graphic design skills. I could not have done this without you.

CONTENTS

Foreword..i

Introduction iii

    Parallels between Aviation and Surgery ix

Chapter 1 – Authority Gradient 1

Chapter 2 – Non-Technical Skills 20

    Part A – Situational Awareness...20

    Part B – Decision making...33

    Part C – Leadership 44

    Part D – Teamwork...49

    Part E – Communication..54

    Part F – Threat and Error Management...........................61

Chapter 3 – Dealing with Technology.....................68

    Part A – Training..68

    Part B – Understanding new systems...............................72

    Part C – Support services..75

Chapter 4 – Use of Checklists................................79

Chapter 5 – Quick Reference Checklists 85

Conclusion...90

References 98

FOREWORD

In 1977, on a small island in the North Atlantic Ocean just off the west African coast, a number of events occurred which resulted in two heavily loaded Boeing 747 'jumbo' jets colliding on a remote runway killing 583 people. It was, and still is, the worst aviation disaster of all time.

This accident sent shock waves through the aviation community and lead to a massive change in pilot training and crew management focus.

Modern flight crew are now trained not only in physically flying the aircraft whilst managing the enormously complex technologies and systems that new generation aircraft possess, commonly referred to as 'technical skills', but their training also encompasses 'non-technical' aspects of human behaviour.

Why do we react the way we do under certain circumstances and pressures?

How do we make decisions?

How do we communicate effectively with each other and how do we perceive and understand the ever-changing environment around us?

These are some of the 'Human Factors' aspects that now form a large part of pilot training.

Is it possible that other areas of expertise and professions could benefit from this type of human behavioural training?

Could the tragic and extremely costly lessons learned by aviation over the years provide opportunities for the wider community to enhance their current work practices?

What does aviation and surgery have in common?

'Ladies and Gentlemen, this is your Surgeon speaking' explores these parallels between the worlds of aviation and surgery and hopefully gives relevance to the concept of the 'Human Factor' in both environments.

INTRODUCTION

Firstly, many thanks for having the curiosity to pick up this book!

It is this sense of curiosity that I hope will continue throughout our journey together as we examine the parallels of our respective professional worlds.

All I ask is that you keep an open mind throughout, a mind that can explore the concepts in this book and examine possibilities of using this knowledge in your daily professional practice.

I must start however but stating very clearly what this book *isn't*.

I never want you to think that I am trying to tell you how to manage your operating theatres, medical practices etc. This is NOT a 'How To' instruction manual!

Nor am I expressing judgement of any kind on current surgical practice and/or expertise in any way.

There is however, value in learning from each other's experience and it's my very great hope that you may find something in the aviation experiences outlined here that you could apply to your working environment, wherever and whatever you may be practicing.

This book also does not, in any way, cast judgment on any of the aviation incidents and accidents, and the people involved contained herein, but merely uses them to highlight certain human traits, shortcomings and behaviours etc. to further explore the value of those lessons being used elsewhere.

Aviation has learned many such lessons, often at a terrible human cost, lessons which deserve to be heeded by not just the aviation world, but by all professions that attempt to ensure the safest outcomes for those in their care.

We will explore in depth these events and discuss the possible learning applications in other areas while also exploring the potential parallels with surgery, medical practice and aviation.

So, what are my qualifications to write such a book?

Currently, I am a Training Captain with a major international airline. I have been flying for over thirty years having had the privilege of flying such aircraft as the Boeing 767, 747 (Classic and 400 series) 787 Dreamliner and the Airbus A330. The training world has been part of my flying career for over 18 years and has been a wonderful journey as pilot training continues to evolve from the technical, hands on act of flying an aircraft, to the non- technical, or 'Human Factors' arena. Large commercial aircraft require a highly developed management structure to stay on top of complex aircraft systems and rapidly accelerating technology whilst also ensuring effective crew utilisation.

Prior to the airlines, I flew in general aviation in remote areas of far north Queensland and the Northern Territory. I have seen some incredible sights, met a diverse and enlightened group of aviators and passengers, and learnt much about myself along the way.

I've heard it said that you start your flying career with an empty bag of experience and a full bag of luck. The secret to survival in aviation is to fill the bag of experience before emptying the bag of luck!

It was a very good grounding for me; operating in an environment with little in the way of support facilities, no radar, no autopilots, no GPS! etc. with the plane fuelled, checked and loaded all by one person. Me.

Through this experience I discovered much about my personal reactions to pressure; how I behaved in various situations, engine and system failures, dwindling daylight approaching outback airstrips with no aerodrome lighting and the like. Having to improvise with the little I had available. I didn't realise it at the time, but my study of human factors and behaviour had already begun whilst flying a range of aircraft in various states of airworthiness in extreme outback conditions.

The connection to the health sciences, came through my general nursing training at the Royal North Shore Hospital in Sydney in the late seventies, well before I learnt to fly.

Back then, nursing was hospital based rather than in a tertiary institution. My training included rotations through the operating theatre, intensive care and general ward areas.

After my general nursing training, I specialized in paediatric intensive care at the Royal Children's' hospital in Camperdown. I have also had surgical experience assisting in ENT, ophthalmology and general theatre work.

My observations in this book therefore come from a background in both aviation and nursing, coupled with a passion for education, particularly in the area of human behaviour, or simply put, 'why people do what they do.'

I've seen massive changes in technology, automation and navigation systems, not to mention crew changes as some of these jobs have been phased out due new technology.

For example, the flight deck used to be crewed by a Captain, First Officer, Second Officer, Radio Operator, Navigator and Flight Engineer. Modern flight decks now are normally crewed by only the Captain and First Officer. Second Officers are carried when the flights are over a certain flight time. The Radio Operator, Navigator and Flight Engineer are gone, as the pilots, using modern technologies perform these tasks themselves.

Nursing, flying and a fascination for human behaviour has led to me presenting to many surgical teams on behalf of various sponsors over the past few years, specifically dealing with some of these questions…

- Can surgery/medicine benefit from the lessons learnt in aviation?
- Are there parallels between Aviation and Surgery?
- What can both areas of expertise learn from each other?
- What areas of Human Factors training currently being utilized by pilots could be used by surgical teams and or other areas of medical practice?

And so, after many of these presentations, getting incredibly positive, often robust, lively interaction and feedback from many different areas of surgery and medicine both during and after the presentations, I decided to expand the content of my presentations into this book.

It is my very great hope that, within the stories and examples presented in these pages, you may be able to identify concepts and/or techniques that you will be able to use in your practice and that areas of expertise outside of the aviation sphere in general can benefit from the experiences, lessons and current training that exist in the aviation world.

For convenient referral or refresher of the various chapters, I've included a summary of 'checklists' that covers the main questions posed by the chapter content. We pilots call such a summary a "Quick Reference

Handbook' or QRH. Hopefully you will refer back to certain chapters by using the 'QRH' as a refresher.

I sincerely hope you enjoy 'Ladies and Gentlemen, this is your Surgeon speaking' and look forward to any feedback you may have.

PARALLELS BETWEEN AVIATION AND SURGERY

So, what are the parallels between the flight deck and the operating theatre?

- Both Aviation and Surgery use teams comprising of various expertise levels, designated into defined roles using many different skill sets.
- Both have a defined structure or 'Authority Gradient'. (more on this later).

On the flight deck is the Captain, the First Officer and the Second Officer.

The operating theatre team contains Specialist surgeons, usually their Surgical Registrar, Residents, Anaesthetist, scrub nurses, scout nurses and often ancillary technicians and life support staff. (in no particular order)

- Both strive to achieve the safest possible outcome for those in our care.
- Both Aviation and Surgery utilise the services of human beings and, like it or not, we humans are subject to various conditions such as fatigue, distraction, physiological impairment etc. all of which may have an impact on our cognitive and

motor skills. Some of these issues we have little control over e.g. we can't be assured of perfect health every time we're engaging in complex tasks! If we're aware of it, we might have some level of control over other factors, such as realising that fatigue is affecting team performance and it's time for a break.

'Human Factors' therefore apply to any group of humans attempting to complete a task, including situational awareness (or a clear overview of all factors affecting the operation), decision making, teamwork, leadership and communication skills.

How all these human facets are then affected by external influences, team dynamics, environmental conditions and fatigue levels is an area of great interest when it comes to studying teams of professionals at work.

Distraction is another issue altogether. Sometimes it takes the form of focusing on unrelated things (I have seen cases of pilots busily talking on their mobiles, dealing with domestic issues instead of attending to correctly configuring the aircraft during pre-flight procedures). At other times, it may be a prioritisation concern, when a less important issue takes precedence over a more crucial one. There have been cases of flight crews being so focused on dealing with a technical abnormality that they have run out of fuel before landing! As unlikely as this sounds, it comes down to someone maintaining the 'BIG picture'. (more about this later).

Medical staff can be distracted simply because they have more than one patient to deal with at a time, often with rapidly changing conditions and states of stability. Prioritisation skills must then be called upon to decide which patient is in the most critical need of attention, while keeping a running mental list of all the others!

I conducted a series of recurrent flight checks in the simulator on a particular pilot (the instrument rating proficiency check we have every three months or so) and found him to be a very competent operator. On one occasion however, his performance was way below par, completely out of character for the normal operating standard of this individual.

In the tea break, I took him aside and gently asked him if everything was ok? Everything was ok, he assured me, except for the fact that his wife had walked out on him the night before.

"So why did you even come in today?" I asked.

"Well, I just wanted to get the check ride out of way, so I didn't have something else to worry about."

I gently suggested that he might want to think about going home and take some time out to attend to his present situation. Sometimes we underplay the effect these external issues have, taking up valuable 'hard drive space' in our heads, making it difficult to think through the emotional fog.

- Both Aviation and Surgery make use of technologies that are advancing at an ever-increasing pace. These technologies bring about their own series of challenges so that we can use the equipment effectively and safely while keeping ahead of the changes. This is discussed in depth in a later chapter.

At the end of the day, the best and safest outcome for those in our care is our ultimate objective. Life however, tends to conjure up situations that make this objective all the more challenging.

1: AUTHORITY GRADIENT

What do I mean by 'authority gradient'?

Basically, it's the old term 'chain of command'. But what it infers is more like a way to describe the general 'flow' of responsibility, decision making and communication along that chain of command.

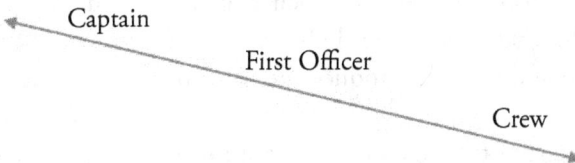

Captain

First Officer

Crew

Let's face it, the buck has to stop somewhere with someone ultimately responsible for the outcome of the operation.

But if the *angle* of the authority gradient between the team members is too steep, it might mean that communication or information flow is stifled or impeded because team members don't feel comfortable verbalizing concepts, concerns or other constructive input to team members further up the chain.

An authority gradient that is flatter or sloping in the opposite direction might mean the head of the team could potentially be overrun with seemingly 'helpful' suggestions, plans and other information, that possibly could engulf his or her sense of overall authority and effectiveness as team leader.

The questions therefore are, do we really need an authority gradient at all and, if so, what is the optimum gradient?

The most effective gradient seems to be the one where no doubt exists as to who the team leader is, that allows for mutual respect for the credentials and experience of the team members but still acknowledges that the head of the team has the ultimate responsibility for the final decisions/outcomes etc. Such a gradient usually has a leader that utilizes the skills, experience and ideas of the team and tends to produce the best possible results.

To ensure the gradient is optimum for any given task, the team leader/Surgeon/Captain needs to provide an atmosphere of open communication where other team members feel comfortable to give input whilst being aware of not stepping over the line and taking over. This balancing act does not come easily, particularly if the team leader is new to the role and acutely feels the weight of responsibility on them. This alone can produce a steepening of the authority gradient, as the leader struggles to feel comfortable and confident in the new role as head of operations and thus carrying the burden of responsibility.

I can vividly remember that exact feeling when I was finally promoted to the rank of Captain, after what seemed like endless simulator and flight assessments. Yes, it's fabulous being the Captain (your jokes are now always funny, you never get the wrong fuel order, and you always get your choice of crew meal…) but the realization soon hits that YOU are responsible for the safety of your crew, hundreds of passengers, the aircraft, other aircraft around you, and of course yourself! So, it's not uncommon for some people, under the weight of this new role, to get very 'serious' for a while until they become comfortable with it. During this time, it could be possible for the authority gradient to become steeper than optimum.

Sound familiar? How did you feel when you first checked out in a higher role, responsibility etc.?

Carrying the weight of ultimate responsibility and feeling comfortable and confident assuming the ownership of your flight deck or operating theatre doesn't come easily or naturally at first.

Establishing an effective authority gradient however, one that reflects your personal management style, is absolutely key to achieving that 'Command confidence'.

I'll never forget something a crusty old Jumbo Captain told me when I was a young Second Officer. I'd flown with some really bad-tempered Captains for the past few trips, but this man was a gentleman. He was respectful, quiet but still very much aware of what was happening. I asked him "Captain, how come you seem so relaxed on the flight deck?" He replied "Son, 99% of the time, this operation runs smoothly without me interfering. I'll speak up if I'm needed for the other 1%".

Providing an atmosphere where all team members are comfortable to give input, share concerns, ideas etc. is so important, it's actually written into our administration policy manuals to "create and maintain an environment where other flight crew members feel confident in expressing concerns about the conduct of the flight without fear of adverse consequences."

Such an optimum gradient as described above also provides a non-threatening work environment thus allowing team members to work to their best potential.

So why do we need this authority gradient at all? Surely the most experienced pilot/doctor or whoever, is the best person to be in charge and run the show, aren't they? Why would they need to be questioned about things at all? Do we all make so many errors as bumbling humans that we have to be constantly covering for each other?

Aside from the obvious fact that human beings are fallible and capable of oversight and/or error at the best of times, the most important reason for providing an effective angle to the authority gradient is to guard against *subtle incapacitation*. Now I'm not talking about the big dramatic convulsion or heart attack in the heat of battle, but a situation that could involve a much less obvious condition like a blood sugar level anomaly or slight stroke, cardiac or gastro-intestinal issue, where the team leader may not even be aware that his or her performance is being adversely affected.

(This is also a strong case for the use of checklists but more about this later…)

To guard against these potentially life-threatening situations, there MUST be a mechanism whereby the team can relay concern, and act appropriately to prevent an undesirable situation from occurring.

Our flight crews are regularly trained in dealing with pilot incapacitation. This forms part of our recurrent training in the flight simulator when one pilot (through a discreet interphone line) is told to stop responding to the other pilots calls or other inputs. The remaining pilot has to then ensure (sometimes using the cabin crew to help) that the sick pilot is not obstructing the flight controls (there's been actual cases of pilots having epileptic type seizures and pushing violently on the rudder pedals…) and then taking control of the aircraft and conducting the approach and landing on his or her own.

Our co-pilots are also trained in the use of "Emergency Language" which, put simply, is a structure that can be used where necessary to express concern to the Captain about the state of flight if required. If no appropriate response to the question is received, after increasing levels of concern have been expressed, the First officer may actually assume Command and take over the aircraft.

This structure is to mitigate the risk of subtle incapacitation affecting flight crew.

There have been many aircraft accidents caused by pilot incapacitation where there was no communication of any kind from the other crew members on the flight deck heard on the Cockpit Voice Recorder (CVR; this constantly records the previous 30 minutes of flight, used in conjunction with the flight data recorder to help accident investigators determine the cause of accidents). Whether those accidents were caused by a lack of training, cultural differences or simply a very steep authority gradient is unclear.

As a Captain, when things get tough, I want and expect 100% effort and commitment from my team. The most effective way to ensure that this will happen consistently, is to provide an open, honest, positive and respectful environment that encourages each member to operate at their optimum potential.

Ketchikan, Alaska. April 5, 1976.

Alaska Airlines Flight 60 was a Boeing 707 arriving at Ketchikan airport, Alaska in winter. The Captain was the pilot flying supported by his First Officer and Flight Engineer. Snow had recently been ploughed from the runway surface and 'braking action' (a term to describe the effectiveness of the brakes in slippery conditions. It is usually reported by other pilots using that runway) had been reported as poor.

Reports tell of the aircraft flying low and fast supposedly to break free of cloud and conduct a visual approach instead of the more time-consuming instrument procedure.

The aircraft landed too fast for the icy conditions and, once the Captain realized the aircraft wasn't going to stop on the remaining runway, even after he had selected reverse thrust, he elected to attempt a 'go around' or aborted landing. Once reverse thrust has been selected on any landing roll, a go around is not an option as there is not enough time for the reverse thrust sleeve panels to retract and the engines to fully develop forward take-off power.

The cockpit voice recorder clearly indicates that the First Officer expressed concern about both the low approach altitude and the high energy state of the aircraft on approach.

This information was not only disregarded by the Captain, but also used as a source of ridicule by both the Captain and the Flight Engineer! Now I know this is an extreme example of a complete lack of effective cockpit resource management, but it is certainly indicative of how far aviation has come in learning from this type of behaviour.

The following is a section of the transcript of the cockpit voice recorder...

First Officer	Want me to fly today?
Captain	No Response
First Officer	What's the glide slope there John?
Captain	Well, we know where we are … we'll be alright
Flight Engineer	Don't you worry, the fox is gonna have it wired.
First Officer	I hope so.
Captain	No problem.
First Officer	This a little faster than you normally fly this, John?
Captain	Oh yeah, but it's nice and smooth. We're gonna get in right on time, maybe a little ahead of time. We got it made.
First Officer	Sure hope so.
Flight Engineer	You know John, what's the difference between a duck and a co-pilot?
Captain	What is that?
Flight Engineer	A duck can fly.
Captain	Well said.
First Officer	Seems like there's a bit of tail wind up here, John.
Captain	Yeah, we're savin gas …help us get in a couple of minutes early too.
First Officer	John, you're just a little below the MDA (maximum descent altitude) here.
Captain	Yeah, we'll take care of it here.
First Officer	This is a little too high.
Captain	Yeah, gear down.
First Officer	You really look awfully high.
Captain	15 degree flaps … 25 on the flaps.

First Officer	John, you're really high …you're gonna need 40 on the flaps here to get this thing down. I don't think you're gonna make it John, if you don't get this sucker on the ground.
Flight Engineer	Get it down, John.
First Officer	I don't think you're gonna make it. I don't think you're gonna make it.
Captain	We're going around. Oh darn.
Flight Engineer	130, 140 knots.
First Officer	It isn't gonna stop John. We're not gonna make it John. Great John. I told you. …Geez…

One person died and 32 people were injured.

The authority gradient was so steep that even, though concern was being expressed by a crew member, it was not being considered as pertinent or relevant. Kudos to the First Officer who, even in the face of ridicule, continued to express his doubts about a successful arrival.

Later reports indicated that the Captain had a history of blood sugar anomalies on previous tests, had not eaten for 12 hours prior to the accident and had markedly decreased hearing on audiometry. It is unclear as to whether he was hearing the first officers' concerns, and/or unable to cognitively process the information in a timely manner.

I remember a flight a few years ago on a Boeing 767 from Tokyo to Sydney, scheduled to leave just before they closed the airport at 2300 local time due to curfew.

As we prepared the aircraft for takeoff, one of the flight attendants in the aft galley called to report a strange smell, one that he'd never experienced before.

The ground engineer had a quick trip to the aft galley and reported nothing unusual and suggested that the aircraft was ok to depart.

Ground staff were keen to get us going as they didn't want the problem of finding 200 hotel rooms in Tokyo at short notice if we missed curfew time of 2300!

Pressure was mounting to leave, all the while, the nagging doubt and the flight attendants report still persisted in my mind.

I sent the Second Officer down there for a second opinion. He reported a slight odour but had no idea of the origin. Meanwhile the flight attendant was adamant that it was something he hadn't encountered. To cut a long story short, we insisted on engineering trouble shooting the immediate area for any form of electrical burning etc. finally discovering a potable water pump, which sits above the rear left-hand toilet cubicle, was electrically shorting out and actually melting in its housing, with the fumes going into the ventilation system near the aft galley!

Now the flight attendants may or may not have the engineering knowledge to trouble shoot these things, but when they say they'd never smelt something like that before, after years of flying, I listened!

The smouldering remnants of the pump were quickly removed, the area secured, and we departed 5 minutes before curfew.

Now, while I'm not banging my own leadership drum here, I was glad that the cabin crew felt comfortable enough to report something as vague as the initial signs early on in the pre-flight. Had the authority gradient been too steep, they might not have given us this crucial information or, we may have completely disregarded it. Tokyo to Sydney at night, flying over all that water with a melting potable water pump is not a pleasant prospect!

In a study conducted by the USA's National Transport Safety Board of US Carriers accidents between 1978 and 1995, it was found that 80% of accidents occurred when the Captain was the flying pilot. Only 20% occurred when the First officer was the flying pilot. Did that mean that First officers were better pilots than Captains? Or did it mean that the First Officers, in their duty as non-flying pilot or 'pilot monitoring' as we now refer to it, were more reluctant to point out errors to the Captain than the other way around?

Even the term 'non-flying pilot' was thought to be too passive and, in an attempt to increase vigilance on the flight deck, the role was renamed 'pilot monitoring'

I often ask my audiences in my surgical presentations if they, working as a junior staff member, have ever seen a less than desirable technique being used or decision being made with no comment or concern raised by the rest of the team members during a procedure? The responses are very interesting indeed.

After speaking with a surgeon recently however, it seems that the medical, surgical authority gradient may not be as clear cut as the flight deck.

He was saying that often, there are multiple specialties in the same operating theatre, but rarely is there a discussion about who is the overall team leader. In a crisis, usually someone rises to the leadership level, and it may depend on what sort of crisis that will determine the leadership roles e.g. if the nature of the crisis is predominately surgical, then a surgeon may become team leader, on the other hand, if the crisis is anaesthetic in nature, then the anaesthetist might be in charge. However, this is not always the case as sometimes a surgical crisis requires the anaesthetist to be the team leader, because the surgeon must focus on a technical skill or is at risk of becoming task saturated. There are also situations where a surgical registrar might be the most senior surgeon in the room, but the anaesthetist is the most senior doctor in the room if they are a consultant.

This variability in team structure certainly muddies the authority gradient waters!

Does there need to be some form of discussion in cases where there are multiple specialties involved as to who has total oversight and responsibility for the operation, who is responsible for coordinating the various specialities, and who is in charge of it all goes pear shaped?

So, when examining your own situation, what's the angle of the authority gradient in your workplace environment?

Is it always clearly defined, or, as we saw in the previous example, does it have a variability about the overall structure? How do various teams cope with this change of leadership on a daily basis?

Would your team members feel comfortable expressing concerns or just generally giving constructive input?

Have you ever discussed strategies to combat the possibility of subtle incapacitation?

Another example where a steep authority gradient may have contributed to an accident occurred in the Canary Islands.

Tenerife, Canary Islands. March 27, 1977.

In 1977, a bomb exploded in the airport terminal at Gran Canaria airport in the Canary Islands, off the coast of Morocco.

Aircraft inbound to Los Palmas airport on Gran Canaria had to divert to other places as the runway there was closed for inspection and repairs. Most of the traffic diverted to Los Rodeos airport on the island of Tenerife.

Now, Los Rodeos wasn't used to heavy airline traffic and the small runway and taxiways weren't setup to handle this amount of traffic.

The airport itself is elevated nearly 600m above sea level and is subject to poor visibility due to low level cloud formations.

When things don't go according to the original plan like that, it puts huge pressure on flight crew due to their limited flight duty hours. It varies from country to country, but basically there are limits to the tour of duty that pilots can operate under, usually extendable under certain circumstances, but only to a point. Breaking these regulations is prohibited and, in a case like an unexpected diversion, the pressure mounts to re-fuel the aircraft and get ready for another departure, all within legal tour of duty limits.

Two aircraft were in exactly that situation, a KLM Royal Dutch Airlines 747, KLM 4805 and a Pan American World Airways 747, Pan Am 1736. Both sets of crews were keen to refuel and be ready as soon as Los Palmas airport opens again.

Pan Am 1736 was actually first to be ready, but was blocked by KLM who was still refuelling, deciding to put on extra fuel to save time back at Gran Canaria airport.

When KLM was eventually ready, the weather started closing in, with visibility reducing dramatically as a type of sea fog rolled in.

Due to the limited taxiways available at Tenerife, and to save time, Air Traffic Control instructed KLM 747 to taxi down the runway itself, with the expectation that he would do a 180 degree turn at the end to line up in the takeoff position.

The Pan Am 747 was also cleared to taxi behind KLM on the runway but instructed to take the third taxiway to the left and report clear of the runway.

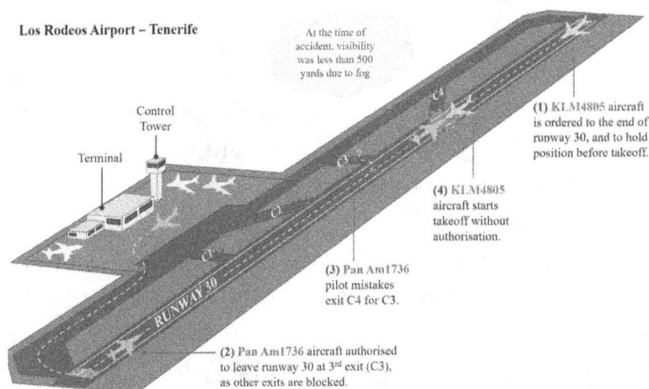

Los Rodeos Airport – Tenerife

At the time of accident, visibility was less than 500 yards due to fog

Control Tower

Terminal

RUNWAY 30

(1) KLM4805 aircraft is ordered to the end of runway 30, and to hold position before takeoff.

(4) KLM4805 aircraft starts takeoff without authorisation.

(3) Pan Am1736 pilot mistakes exit C4 for C3.

(2) Pan Am1736 aircraft authorised to leave runway 30 at 3rd exit (C3), as other exits are blocked.

All this time the visibility was such that the ground controller couldn't see either aircraft and was relying solely on VHF radio communications to implement the plan.

One problem with VHF radio though, is only one person can transmit at a time. It's not a 'party line system' so if two people transmit at the same moment, a static hissing sound is the only sound that anyone can hear.

Here's where it gets messy. The KLM 747 performs a 180 degree turn at the end of the runway to get in position to take-off, and the Captain goes to advance the throttles when the First Officer states that they do not have an ATC clearance.

"I know that, ask" replies the Captain and a departure clearance (heading and altitude instructions to be flown '*after* takeoff') was issued on the VHF radio by ATC.

Because the word "takeoff" was used in the clearance by ATC, the KLM crew thought that included a clearance to take off as well. Trouble with that concept however was that the Pan AM 747 was still taxiing down the same runway trying to find the third taxiway so that they can get clear of the runway!

Here's the crucial point where the 'non-routine' issues of that unusual day come together. Visibility reducing, limited ATC services (where English is not their first spoken language) VHF radios capable of blocking transmissions if they occur simultaneously, and crew keen to get going to avoid exceeding flight duty time limitations, all coming together toward disaster.

The KLM Captain announced "We gaan" (or "we are going") and advanced the throttles for takeoff believing he had a clearance to do so.

Tenerife ATC responded with "OK, standby for takeoff, I will get back to you." ('OK' not being standard phraseology in aviation).

After this exchange, the Pan AM First Officer tried to transmit to the tower to say that they were still taxiing down the runway, with ATC responding...

"Roger, report when clear".

This exchange prompted the KLM First Officer and Flight Engineer to verbalize something like "so he's not clear then?" or words to that effect to which the KLM Captain firmly announced "Jawal" (Yes).

The rest, as they say is history, with the Pan AM jumbo crew seeing the KLM aircraft coming at them out of the mist and trying valiantly to get out of the path of the oncoming aircraft.

They collided just as the KLM 747 got airborne and 583 people died in the fiery crash of the two aircraft.

The Captain of the KLM aircraft was their Senior Training Captain and had featured on many KLM inflight publications. He had spent the previous six months in the flight simulator training other pilots but hadn't had a lot of 'real time' flight hours leading up to that event.

It's obvious from this horrific event, that many factors were at play for it to end so tragically. Perhaps if the weather hadn't closed in, so both the aircraft and the tower had 'the big picture' (more about this concept later) or if the KLM 747 hadn't put on extra fuel thus carrying the extra weight, it might have cleared the PAN AM aircraft on takeoff.

If the other KLM crew had expressed concern that they hadn't been cleared for takeoff, the Captain may have paused to confirm with the tower that takeoff clearance.

If, if, if….

So, what could other professional teams possibly learn from this event? Up until this accident and following another one in 1978 involving an aircraft that ran out of fuel while attempting to diagnose a landing gear problem, aviation hadn't really focused on human related factors, concerning leadership, teamwork, decision making, situational awareness and communication. These initial aspects were known as "Crew Resource Management" or CRM and continues today as a large part of flight training.

Given that the 'big picture' was somewhat hazy in the Tenerife accident, would it be feasible to suggest that many varying factors are involved in day to day surgery too? Team dynamics closed or effective communication, long surgical lists, fatigue levels among the team, distraction etc. are some factors that possibly could have an impact on performance.

Who has and maintains 'the big picture'?

Does technology get in the way or enhances the maintenance of 'the big picture'?

Remember, I'm simply asking the questions as food for thought here, not supplying the answers!

There was a question in the Tenerife accident, that the "cockpit gradient" was too steep for the other crew to feel comfortable to challenge the Captain. Is it possible that surgical teams might experience and similar phenomenon and not be willing to give input, for a variety of reasons, when things aren't going so well?

What is the angle of your authority gradient?

2: NON-TECHNICAL SKILLS

Part A – Situational Awareness

One of the key skills required by pilots is the constant maintenance of 'Situational Awareness' (SA), often referred to as keeping the 'big picture'.

Sounds simple, doesn't it? Like anything that sounds simple though, it's often the exact opposite when faced with the ever-changing status of complex situations.

The definition often used for situational awareness in an aviation sense is…

"The monitoring of progress and overall management to allow accurate perception of all factors affecting the aircraft and crew"

Situational awareness is made up of three levels…

- Perception;
- Understanding; and
- Anticipation.

The majority of operational errors experienced by flight crew originally stem from a lack of accurate and/or appropriate perception of available information.

It follows that levels of understanding may also be affected by this perceptive shortfall, thus leading to a reduced ability to anticipate new events.

The paradox of situational awareness in a nutshell, is that you don't realize you've lost it, because you don't have it!

When we train our flight crews in the flight simulator, we focus on developing strategies to maintain situational awareness (workload management, load shedding, control of operational pace...) and to recognise signs of potentially losing situational awareness in both yourself and/or your crew.

The flight simulator is used with great effect here, using high workload and complex technical events to give the crew practice in these techniques whilst under pressure, and to give them a chance to 'feel', while in a safe and controlled environment, what it's like to be overwhelmed and lose situational awareness. If pilots are aware of this feeling, they are more likely to recognise it, intervene earlier and regain control.

Often sessions are recorded on video and segments replayed to allow crew to assess their own ability to maintain situational awareness.

It is not unrealistic to suggest that we each perceive things differently. Maintenance of situational awareness as a team requires clear and open analysis of information to guard against each crewmember having their own version of the 'big picture'.

The other side of the coin is a phenomenon known as 'group think' where a team convinces one another that one particular perception of information is correct. This can occur when one personality type dominates less confident individuals, or the 'authority gradient' is too steep for effective communication and overall team vision to exist.

It is imperative that crew have a chance to analyse information independently before conferring, to minimize 'group think', coupled with a supportive working environment (shallow gradient) in which they feel confident to express their opinion.

Cali, Colombia. December 20, 1995.

In 1995 an American Airlines Boeing 757 left Miami Florida for Cali in Colombia. Both flight crew members were highly experienced on both the aircraft type and operations to South America.

Weather enroute and at the destination was mainly fine.

The departure from Miami however was nearly two hours late due to late arriving connecting passengers.

The flight crew were scheduled for 'minimum rest' in Cali, as specified by their flight crew duty limit restrictions, and were worried that this initial delay would affect the timing of their departure the following day.

The First Officer was the pilot flying while the Captain was communicating with Air Traffic Control and managing the FMS or Flight Management System. The FMS is a series of computers responsible for navigation and flight parameter management such as speed schedules, enroute navigation and fuel predictions.

The flight progressed uneventfully until approaching descent.

Given the forecast wind direction at Cali, the crew anticipated the approach would take them southbound, over the top of the airfield and then land into wind back toward the north. This approach had been loaded into the FMS.

Cali is also a non-radar environment, where ATC relies on the aircraft reporting at various points so that they can provide separation from other aircraft.

The crew commenced a descent profile based on the expected approach but were then asked by ATC if they could accept a landing 'straight in' towards the south as the wind at the field was now calm. This would result in less track miles flown, quicker flight time and would help minimise the delay. The problem was however, that their altitude was very high for this change of approach and they had very little time to program, brief and fly this 'unexpected' change to the aircraft's flight path.

The First Officer stated on the cockpit voice recorder "We'll have to scramble to get down. We can do it."

The crew were then cleared to fly direct to a navigation beacon called 'Rozo' and to report passing another navigation beacon called Tulua 21 nautical miles from the airfield at 5,000 ft.

They entered the letter 'R' into the FMS and that bought up a list of points with 'R' as the designator (normally the top one on the list is the closest one to the aircraft) and selected the top 'R' on the list to navigate the aircraft to that point. The problem here though was that the Rozo beacon is actually labelled 'ROZO' as two beacons cannot have the same identifier in the same country. The point they selected was actually Bogota some 130 nautical miles from their position and in a different direction. The selected beacon was not part of Cali airport arrival patterns at all.

The aircraft was now gently banking left toward Bogota, turning some 18 degrees off the original heading and still descending, now into mountainous terrain.

The flight crew were busy finding new charts and re-briefing the new approach all while attempting to lose height faster than a normal descent by extending the aircraft speed brakes (large panels on the upper surface of the wing that reduce lift causing it to descend faster).

Minutes later, the crew became aware that the aircraft was not heading in the required direction. The cockpit voice recorder indicated a confused discussion between the pilots as to the position of the aircraft. The fact that ATC could not help them to resolve the dilemma by a radar position fix made the situation even more complex.

The aircraft then descended into an area of high mountainous terrain as the pilots were attempting to get back onto their original track towards the airport.

Eventually the Ground Proximity Warning System (GPWS) was heard on the cockpit voice recorder ordering the pilots to "PULL UP". They carried out the terrain avoidance manoeuvre but the speed brakes, previously deployed to rapidly lose height, were still extended during the terrain escape manoeuvre.

The aircraft hit the terrain and all 151 passengers and 8 crew members were lost.

ATC reported later that they were confused by the pilots' requests for navigational assistance as their English language proficiency was limited.

Somewhere along the line the big picture was obscured and attempts to regain it were unsuccessful. As with most aviation events, multiple causal factors were identified; unexpected change of approach clearance, non-radar environment, high terrain, multiple similar navigation beacons in the same area, commercial pressures to minimize delays, to name a few.

Portland, Oregon. December 28, 1978.

In 1978 a DC-8 aircraft inbound to Portland experienced a landing gear malfunction on final approach. They decided to discontinue that approach to allow trouble shooting. The cause of the landing gear warning light indication remained unknown despite remedial checklist action.

The crew then went on to prepare the aircraft for a potential emergency landing on the remaining landing gear, giving the cabin crew and passengers a full briefing on their expectations of the landing and emergency drills to follow.

The Captain wanted to give the cabin as much time to prepare for this emergency and regularly checked on their progress. The cabin crew said that they required more time to prepare, which they were given. The aircraft was in a holding pattern while these preparations were carried out.

After all cabin preparations were thoroughly completed, the flight crew commenced the approach. During the approach, they noticed the engines were failing due to fuel starvation and there wasn't enough fuel remaining to fly to the runway and land. The aircraft crashed short of the runway in an area of trees.

Somewhere along the track, the big picture (including monitoring *all* factors affecting the operation, including the fuel status) was lost and the crew became task focused on getting the cabin ready for the landing.

- So, who is responsible for maintaining situational awareness in the operating theatre environment? (who has and maintains the big picture?)
- How is the perception of new data affecting the procedure shared with all team members to ensure the big picture is a common vision? (also referred to as the 'shared mental model')
- How are changes to the individual situations communicated to the rest of the team, anaesthetic staff, life support technicians, nursing staff etc. to ensure everyone's on the same page?
- What factors could impede maintaining good situational awareness?

The list might include, but certainly not limited to, fatigue (long surgical lists), unexpected technical complexity, inexperienced team members, less than optimum 'authority gradient', or simply having a bad day! Let's face it, if we are totally honest with ourselves, there are some days when we are sharper than others...

Another possible impediment is a syndrome known as 'expectation bias' where our perception of a situation is affected by previous experiences and/or expectations.

This could lead us to believe that a situation is similar to something you've dealt with before with successful implementation of one particular technique or the other, only to find however, that you're dealing with something completely different.

- How does the training of medical professionals consider or acknowledge the importance of maintaining situational awareness?
- How do we regain situational awareness once it's been lost?

A surgeon friend of mine recently relayed a story from his early surgical training.

He was a registrar working with a specialist general surgeon performing a cholecystectomy, before laparoscopic technology was available.

The head surgeon was having difficulty identifying a bleeder and was getting increasingly frustrated and anxious. He turned to my friend and said " Well, we'll just have to close up" and started to close the wound. Without any human factors training, my friend recognised a possible loss of situational awareness and simply applied some pressure to the wound site, saying in a calm, non-judgmental way "maybe we just need to step back for a minute and have a think about this. Have a rest. I've got it."

His superior did indeed physically step back from the table, took some deep breaths and regained perspective. He then proceeded to isolate the bleeding vessel, then finished the procedure. The situation needed someone to recognise that things were not proceeding as they should be and have the courage to gently intervene to allow some 'clear air' thinking space.

I believe the key here is clear, effective communication. Either you verbalize that you're having difficulty or confusion with a certain issue or recognise that someone else may be having difficulty coping with something.

Herein lies the problem as no-one wants to admit any sort of failing for fear of judgement by their team or peers! So, it could be a double-edged sword i.e. you've lost the thread and *don't know it*, or you've lost the thread and *won't admit it*.

Someone in the team then needs to slow everything down, get back to basics, seek more information, *rebuild the platform*, reassess and replan.

Realistic, honest self-assessment is crucial in the effective maintenance of situational awareness. If any team member is losing the plot, *including* the Captain/Surgeon, it is vital that this is recognized, communicated and dealt with promptly before things escalate. This admission is *not* a sign of weakness or inability to complete the task to a proficient standard, it's actually the opposite and an action that could prevent greater errors being made.

That action may be as simple as a quick break, pause, or whatever is necessary to regather your thoughts and check that you're still on task and achieving the objective.

As the Captain of the aircraft, I have absolutely no qualms whatsoever in admitting that I don't understand something or I'm not sure which mode of action is appropriate to a given situation. Sometimes things come 'out of left field' and someone in the team might have valuable experience in that particular situation to share. I've flown with some pilots that, in their previous working lives, were aircraft engineers. They possessed invaluable expertise when it came to dealing with a complex problem on board.

Of course, the final decision is always mine, as pilot in command, but I will use all the resources I have available, including my crew, to come to that decision.

This greatly enhances the overall safety of the operation. As previously mentioned however, it's often difficult to pick when the big picture has been lost.

Some signs of this may include task fixation or preoccupation, confusion, communication breakdowns or unexpected departures from standard procedures.

Every situation is different as every individual team member's perceptions and responses are different. Therefore, the remedy for fixing a lapse in situational awareness will depend on the severity and complexity of the situation. The principles of regaining situational awareness however are the same.

Stop, slow down, reassess, re-establish standard procedures, enquire as to the state of other team members "Is anyone else starting to get tired here?"

Its common in the flight simulator to see situations developing their own 'rhythm'.

By this I mean that the operational pace was largely determined by the problem they were facing. Obviously, some situations require expeditious treatment such as engine or cargo fire. Generally, however, the operational pace must be controlled by the flight crew, especially the Captain. If the aircraft is committed to a landing without the appropriate preparation, because the crew have been rushing to get on the ground, things can be missed and safety compromised.

The 'rhythm' of the situation, needs to be managed to allow all procedural steps, checklists etc. to be completed before committing to an approach and landing. This may mean flying one more holding pattern, or getting a radar heading from Air Traffic control or such other strategy.

I was on the last flight of a long tour of duty recently flying from Melbourne to Perth and back. On our descent back into Melbourne, the weather radar was indicating extensive thunderstorm activity around Melbourne airport. Aircraft were attempting to navigate around these storm cells, as they are associated with severe turbulence and possible icing conditions. We were manoeuvring around storm cells and flew over the top of Melbourne airport with the plan of turning left toward the north and eventually landing back to the south on runway 16. After turning north however, the radar indicated more storm activity directly on the approach for that particular runway, making plan 'A' somewhat unattractive!

By this stage our tour of duty was pushing 11 hours. We'd had multiple heading and speed changes and the planned approach was now looking uncertain. I started to feel as if the big picture was becoming cloudy (pun intended) and our situation and available options were not clear cut.

The radar indicated clear skies to the northeast so, after conferring with the First Officer (and communicating my hesitation to committing to the approach at this time), we requested with ATC a heading into the clear and a climb to 5000ft.

We levelled at 5000ft, took a short time out, slowed the aircraft down and turned back toward the Melbourne area, where we both felt the 'big picture' had been restored and could see that the approach toward the runway facing west (runway 27) was relatively clear. After a check on the current wind direction, we told ATC that we required an approach onto that runway.

After landing we discussed our performance and reinforced the necessity to intervene when things weren't going smoothly, take a short break and get some *clear air* in which to plan further.

The other non-technical aspects such as communication, teamwork, leadership and decision-making directly affect the maintenance of sound situational awareness.

If any one of these areas is deficient, it has a direct impact on the effectiveness of the others.

These areas of non-technical behaviour are not limited to the flight deck or operating theatre. They can be applied any time a group of humans interact to achieve a common goal.

What strategies do you have for keeping the big picture?

Have you ever lost it and, if so, how did you get it back? (its ok to admit it, you're reading by yourself!)

Part B – Decision making

Every day we make thousands of decisions. Every procedure, consultation, even driving to work involves some degree of decision making.

So *how* then, do we make decisions?

Is that as ridiculous as it sounds? Don't you just, you know, make them?

Well, some decisions are made just like that, often with little conscious thought. My shoes are undone, I need to tie them up now so I don't trip over. Done.

Breakfast? What do we have? What do I feel like? Done.

But are the decisions made in a complex environment such as the operating theatre or flight deck made so casually?

Basically, there are two types of decision-making processes.

One is an 'Analytical' decision making process, involving a structured, methodical approach to achieving a decision.

This form of decision making is often used in a complex technical environment involving many relevant factors. For example, in aviation, if the crew members are inexperienced on a particular aircraft type or destination, they might prefer a more detailed, methodical approach to decision making.

One such strategy used very effectively in aviation training is the G.R.A.D.E. process where the 'G' stands for gathering information, the 'R' is reviewing that information, 'A' analysing the alternatives, 'D' is deciding on a course of action and 'E' stands for the evaluating that decision.

This method is not meant to be like a linear pipe with a one-way valve...

G R A D E

but a constantly circulating process where more information is sought and investigated and the effectiveness of decisions re-evaluated.

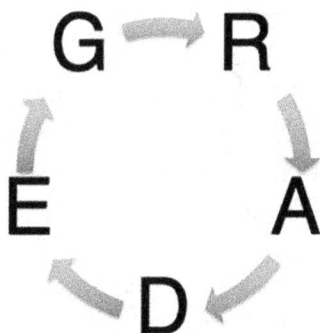

G R
E   A
D

It is commonly seen in pilot training where a sound GRADE process has been followed at the time, but the crew have not been flexible enough to deal with new information resulting in a less than optimum result. It's almost as if, once a decision has been made, it's an admission of defeat or loss of face even, to change it for another course of action even though new information, such as updated weather forecasts, is available.

I've also seen trainees so afraid of making a poor decision that they cannot make any decision at all! The problem with that scenario however is that, as the old saying goes, "Every takeoff is voluntary, every landing is compulsory". You've eventually got to put her down somewhere!

The decision-making progress becomes a continual mini risk assessment, as new information is evaluated and an overall risk re-evaluation occurs along every stage.

Operational confidence comes from the belief that you will make a sound decision based on the information you have available, whilst also regularly reassessing the appropriateness of that decision in the light of any new information forthcoming.

A lot of these management techniques and processes all come down to one particular aspect. It's all about the quality of the questions you're asking!

Asking good quality questions will normally lead to getting better quality answers!

What exactly is the problem? Define it, examine it, check for possible ramifications that could arise. Makes defining the final objective a lot easier.

How much time do I have available? An uncontrollable engine fire on takeoff has a lot less thinking time available than a single electrical generator failure!

Who can help me get more information about this issue?

Could Air Traffic Control, Bureau of Meteorology, Engineering, or other crew members provide any assistance?

What alternatives do we feel more *comfortable* implementing? (sometimes, when you put 'feeling' words like 'comfortable' you'll get a more honest answer from team members!)

After conducting a methodical analytical style decision making process, I ask myself two important questions as the final 'quality control' step in the process.

1) Is this really where I want to take my aircraft? And if yes,
2) Are we ready to do it?

If the answer is no to either of these questions or brings about any uncertainty or discomfort then I won't commit the aircraft to that plan of action until we've reassessed the situation!

The incident involving a Qantas Airbus A380 departing Singapore where a large piece of engine came adrift and took out multiple aircraft systems as it departed the engine casing was an incredibly complex scenario. This event generated many different system failure messages on the aircrafts' maintenance monitoring computer display and required a very methodical approach to prioritising each failure, dealing with the relevant ones, and conducting a safe landing back in Singapore. The crew had to 'think outside the square' as the computerised calculations designed to derive landing distance required in different failure scenarios weren't built to handle so many different system failures at once. The crew had to work with the information they were presented with, adapt quickly to that situation and provide a solution that would result in the safest outcome.

Every element of the crews' human factors training was tested that day and the successful outcome was as a direct result of effective teamwork, decision making, maintenance of situation awareness, leadership and, of course, clear communication.

The other style of decision making is a more intuitive approach based on experience, where actions and decisions are driven by many years of coping with similar situations and/or time does not allow for a long winded, structured analytical method.

A multiple bird strike on both engines soon after takeoff is one such time limited scenario.

Hudson River, New York City. January 15, 2009.

I think we're all familiar with this incident, especially since the movie 'Sully' came out. Personally, I reckon it's one of the best pieces of flying I've ever seen. It is no small decision to land your aircraft in the water on purpose with virtually no 'thinking' time available, just relying on years of experience and a very quick risk assessment involving all available options.

What makes a scenario like this one even more difficult is the fact that, when a critical event confronts us suddenly, our brains are exposed to a phenomenon known as 'startle factor'. Closely akin to the fight or flight response common to most animals, this startle factor gears our bodies up for a rapid, survival driven response. Blood pressure, heart rate, blood sugar levels and respiration rises to give the body the ability to 'physically' act quickly thus increasing the chances of survival against the perceived threat.

The downside to this physiological response is that cognitive thought (not really a big priority for running away from predators…) is impaired, as all that good blood supply is busy in the muscles as they are prepared to run away from predators.

Research shows that cognitive processes could be impaired for anywhere between 30-60 seconds. These pilots did not have the luxury of that amount of time to make a critical decision.

The Airbus A320 took off from LaGuardia airport in January 2009 and, at around 3000ft above sea level, impacted with a flock of Canada geese. This caused a near total loss of engine thrust on both engines due to the ingestion of these large birds into the engine intakes.

With the limited amount of information that the crew had i.e. current height, position, status of the now failed engines and various options suggested by Air Traffic Control, including a return to La Guardia or a possible landing at Teterboro, and even though they would have been probably fighting the physiological effects of the 'startle', the Captain made the decision to ditch the aircraft in the Hudson River.

The transcript of the aircraft's cockpit voice recorder highlights how little time the Captain had to work this problem.

15:27:10	Captain	birds.
15:27:11	First Officer	whoa.
15:27:11	*[sound of thump/thud(s) followed by shuddering sound]*	
15:27:13	*[sound similar to decrease in engine noise/ frequency begins]*	
15:27:14	First Officer	uh oh.
15:27:15	First Officer	we got one rol- both of 'em rolling back.
15:27:18	Captain	ignition, start.
15:27:21	Captain	I'm starting the APU.
15:27:23	Captain	my aircraft.
15:27:24	First Officer	your aircraft.
15:27:28	Captain	get the [Quick Reference Handbook] loss of thrust on both engines.
15:27:32	First Officer	"mayday mayday mayday. uh this is uh Cactus fifteen thirty nine hit birds, we've lost thrust (in/on) both engines we're turning back towards LaGuardia."

15:27:42	Air Traffic Control	ok uh, you need to return to LaGuardia? turn left heading of uh two two zero.
15:27:46	First Officer	two two zero.
15:28:02	First Officer	airspeed optimum relight. three hundred knots. we don't have that.
15:28:05	Captain	we don't.
15:28:05	Air Traffic Control	Cactus fifteen twenty nine, if we can get it for you do you want to try to land runway one three?
15:28:10	Captain	we're unable. we may end up in the Hudson.
15:28:25	First Officer	yeah. the left one's coming back up a little bit.
15:28:31	Air Traffic Control	arright Cactus fifteen forty nine its gonna be left traffic for runway three one.
15:28:35	Captain	unable.
15:28:36	Air Traffic Control	okay, what do you need to land?
15:28:37	First Officer	(he wants us) to come in and land on one three... for whatever.
15:28:46	Air Traffic Control	Cactus fifteen (twenty) nine runway four's available if you wanna make left traffic to runway four.
15:28:49	Captain	I'm not sure we can make any runway. uh what's over to our right anything in New Jersey maybe Teterboro?

15:28:55	Air Traffic Control	ok yeah, off your right side is Teterboro airport.
15:29:02	Air Traffic Control	you wanna try and go to Teterboro?
15:29:03	Captain	yes.
15:29:11	Captain	"this is the Captain brace for impact."
15:29:21	Air Traffic Control	Cactus fifteen twenty nine turn right two eight zero, you can land runway one at Teterboro.
15:29:21	First Officer	is that all the power you got? * (wanna) number one? or we got power on number one.
15:29:25	Captain	we can't do it.
15:29:26	Captain	go ahead, try number one.
15:29:27	Air Traffic Control	kay which runway would you like at Teterboro?
15:29:28	Captain	we're gonna be in the Hudson.
15:29:33	Air Traffic Control	I'm sorry say again Cactus?
15:29:53	Air Traffic Control	Cactus fifteen forty nine radar contact is lost you also got Newark airport off your two o'clock in about seven miles.
15:30:22	Air Traffic Control	Cactus fifteen twenty nine if you can uh....you got uh runway uh two nine available at Newark it'll be two o'clock and seven miles.
15:30:38	Captain	we're gonna brace.

Captain Sullenberger flew a steady, stable approach onto the surface of the Hudson River and all passengers and crew members survived.

The subsequent National Transport Safety Board investigation ruled that the decision to ditch, given all the circumstances was, in fact, the one resulting in the highest probability that the accident would be survivable.

During this investigation, test pilots attempted, in the flight simulator, to replicate the scenario to explore other options. Apparently, only 8 out of 14 attempts resulted in a successful return to land at an airport. Those pilots however, knew the scenario details beforehand, and even though they simulated the time delay combating the issues associated with startle effect (some 35 seconds) before action was taken, the test pilots would not have had the same physiological stress experienced by Captain Sullenberger and his First Officer.

So, in this case, the Captain made the decision based on experience and 'gut instinct' simply because there wasn't time for an extended structured decision-making process.

If you're in the business of caring for the safety and comfort of the general public, both types of decision-making processes involve a mini 'risk assessment' in which the objective is to minimise the risk for the patients/passengers.

Both analytical and intuitive decision-making styles are, in various circumstances, perfectly appropriate.

The problem arises however, when one team member is using one particular decision-making style, based on years of experience and knowledge that potentially the other team members may not possess.

These intuitive decisions may be absolutely appropriate in that particular situation. It doesn't however, allow any form of cross checking or 'quality control' by the rest of the team.

Now I can hear you saying, "well, I don't want every decision I make on the run in my theatre questioned and evaluated!" and I understand that sentiment completely!

The point is however, if decisions are being made without any feedback to the team, even taking the form of simple communication, it takes away a level of protection when guarding against subtle incapacitation. If other team members are struggling to keep the 'big picture' based on decisions made 'on the run' as it were, they may be less inclined to give any input if they are concerned about an aspect of the operation.

Part C – Leadership

Wow, this is a term we often hear, have virtually no day to day feedback about, and yet are expected to display various levels of leadership in our professional and personal lives! What does the term leadership really mean anyway?

One definition I've heard is…

"The ability to influence others and achieve objectives by setting direction, example and a productive working environment."

Other definitions include…

"The capacity and will to rally men and women to a common purpose and the character which inspires confidence" (Maxwell, 1999).

or

"Leadership can involve influencing people by providing purpose, directions and motivation while operating to accomplish the mission and improve the organisation" (brary, 2010).

- What does good leadership look like?
- Are you aware of your impact as a leader day to day?
- Where do we learn to become 'leaders'?

Anyone in charge of a team of people must have certain leadership qualities and skills but what exactly are they?

- Who really cares what sort of a leader I am anyway?
- Does it really make any difference?

I believe the concept of leadership is inextricably linked to the previous chapter on 'Authority Gradient' where so much of your effectiveness as a leader depends on the working environment you set in day to day working life. Your authority in your team should be a given. How you use that authority is another thing indeed....

Discussions on leadership often contain concepts such as being inspirational, motivational, setting a good example by having sound subject knowledge and displaying expert technique, effective awareness of the condition of both the team members and of him/herself.

Regular, accurate assessment of the abilities, limitations, strengths and weaknesses of the team as a whole, is a huge asset for any leader.

I've also heard it said that a leader should 'involve, engage and empower' their team.

All great sounding terms and concepts, but how exactly is it done?

Apollo 13. April 1970.

Few events tell of such astounding leadership as the dramatic journey of Apollo 13.

In April 1970, the Apollo 13 space craft departed Earth for the moon, under the Command of Jim Lovell.

The departure from Earth was largely uneventful until, around three quarters of the way to the moon, they experienced a massive systems failure onboard when the crew were instructed by Houston ground control to 'stir the cryo tanks' as this was a routine inflight task.

This resulted in a huge explosion and rupturing of the number two oxygen tank followed by the failure of number one tank as well. The flow on effect of these system failures also lead to reduced potable water, heating and electrical power.

Suddenly the objective of the mission changed from a successful moon landing for two astronauts, to the safe return to Earth for the three astronauts.

This story is one of incredible leadership from both the Commander of the spacecraft Jim Lovell and the ground-based Flight Director Gene Kranz.

The lack of oxygen, potable water and heating made the Command Module 'Odyssey' virtually uninhabitable for the remainder of the flight. It was decided to use the Lunar Module 'Aquarius' as a lifeboat for the three astronauts until re-entry into the Earths' atmosphere.

This scenario had never been seen or trained for, and, as the journey wore on, other problems arose, such as increasing amounts of CO_2 in the cabin.

Jim Lovell had an unshakeable vision, to get to the moon. Such was the flexibility of his leadership however, when the moon landing was no longer in the picture, the strength of vision for a safe return to Earth for himself and his crew became equally as unshakeable.

The resilience, adaptability and ingenuity shown by these men and their teams hallmarked their leadership. Faced with an increasing amount of complex problems, their faith in their teams allowed them to do the best job possible without overloading individual capabilities.

Lovell and his crew had to completely depower the Command Module and repower it again just before re-entry. This not only had never been done before, but the ground support teams including other astronauts working in the flight simulators at NASA, wrote the procedure in three days. Procedures this complex normally take three months!

Kranz and his team calculated the quickest way back to Earth was to continue on to the moon and use its gravitational force to 'slingshot' Apollo back towards home.

One of the most astounding achievements however was having to make vitally important course corrections using the Lunar Modules' thrusters and only the alignment with the sun for guidance. Again, this had never been attempted! Incorrect course adjustment would result in an unsuccessful re-entry. Despite being cold, hungry and sleep deprived, the crew made these accurate corrections with virtually no technology to support them.

These men had absolute faith in their teams, their ability to adapt, their resilience, all with little room for fear or doubt.

They allowed their team to function, all the while maintaining the vision, guiding and supporting as required.

To me, that sums up leadership in a nutshell.

The rest, as they say, is history.

Hopefully, it's becoming clearer that none of these 'non-technical' skills are stand-alone entities. Effective Leadership would be virtually impossible without the leader having the 'big picture' (SA), or without the ability to make appropriate decisions and communicate these to the team.

Part D – Teamwork

Sioux City, Iowa. July 19, 1989.

The event in Sioux City Iowa in 1989 involving a DC-10 that had lost all hydraulic power and thus all control of the aircrafts' flight controls, is a great example of amazing teamwork in action (not to mention, great leadership and communication as well!).

The DC-10 has three engines, one of which is located on the vertical tailfin. In this event, that particular engine in the tail suffered a massive uncontained failure, meaning that bits of the engine exploded through the engine casing. Some of these pieces severed the hydraulic lines causing all hydraulic systems to fail. Unfortunately, those same hydraulic systems are the ones that power the flight controls!

Suddenly, the aircraft was not responding to the pilots' inputs on the control column, with both the Captain and First Officer struggling to get some form of control over the aircraft.

The plane was now in a right-hand turn and the nose was dropping. Nothing either pilot could do via the control wheel had any effect. The NTSB report summarised the situation as

> *"The airplane was marginally flyable using asymmetrical thrust from engines No. 1 and 3 after the loss of all conventional flight control systems; however, a safe landing was virtually impossible."*

The crew finally reduced engine power on the left engine and increased power to the right engine to stop the turn. This did have some effect in stopping to turn.

On the flight, in the passenger cabin, was a DC-10 flight instructor, Dennis Fitch, who offered to help. He confirmed from the cabin, that the flight controls were, in fact, not moving at all, then proceeded to the flight deck to offer assistance.

While the Captain and First Officer attempted to gain control via their control columns, Fitch took control of the engine thrust, operating the levers left and right to turn and also achieved some pitch (up and down) control by increasing engine power on both (as the engines are under the wing, increasing thrust tends to have a 'nose up' effect on the aircraft).

While this was going on Captain Alfred Haynes was communicating with Air Traffic Control. Captain Haynes kept very calm throughout this situation as evident by this conversation with ATC…

Sioux City Approach: "United Two Thirty-Two Heavy, the wind's currently three six zero at one; three sixty at eleven. You're cleared to land on any runway."

Haynes: "[laughter] Roger. [laughter] You want to be particular and make it a runway, huh?"

Haynes: "Whatever you do, keep us away from the city."

The crew also contacted their maintenance department via radio who informed them that as a failure of all three hydraulic systems was virtually impossible, no procedures had been written to cover it!

With extremely limited control over this huge aircraft carrying 296 people on board, the crew had to now think about landing the aircraft.

They decided to use the landing gear to help slow the aircraft and to cushion the impact. They had no wing flaps available (wing flaps are used to allow the aircraft to slow to landing speed) no speed brake and, apart from manipulation of the engine thrust levers, no flight controls either.

Somehow, through incredible teamwork, communication and just plain skill, they managed to put the aircraft down, whilst traveling at around 400kms per hours instead of the usual approach speed of around 260kms per hour, onto runway 22 at Sioux City.

The right wing impacted the ground and was torn off the fuselage causing the aircraft to flip inverted and come to a stop upside down in a corn field to the right of the runway and burst into flames.

Tragically, 111 people died in the crash, but, incredibly, 185 people survived this near impossible situation.

Although there was over 100 years of flying experience in that cockpit that day, none of the crew had ever practised, or had any experience in handling that particular scenario. CRM or Crew Resource Management was the major tool used to cope with this complete loss of flight controls. Every crew member volunteered input and this high level of effective teamwork resulted in getting that stricken aircraft back on the ground and saved many lives.

'Teamwork' is working together to achieve common objectives.

• How do you build a 'team' atmosphere and why would that be important day to day?

- What aspects do you require to ensure the team functions effectively and consistently?

Open, honest and respectful communication is a pretty good first step.

Providing the environment where people feel comfortable to contribute ideas etc. (there it is again!). This empowers and gives validity to team members.

Support for others, including an awareness of the pressures and challenges other may be experiencing.

Empowering other team members so that they feel free to give you their best work, day in day out.

Resolving conflict in a calm, respectful manner certainly helps grease the teamwork wheels!

- How effectively does your team function?
- If they function really well, why? What makes them a great team?

It's important to acknowledge why things are going well, not just being on the lookout for negatives. This can help to maintain a great team even if you already have one!

- Do you see yourself in the light of a 'team leader' not just the head surgeon or head of a department?
- If you could think of one thing that would enhance teamwork in your workplace, what would it be?

Part E – Communication

Everything else we've discussed so far in terms of being aware of the 'big picture, or situational awareness, to the qualities of leadership, the structure behind decision making and creating effective teamwork is inextricably linked to our next topic.

Communication is the glue that holds the show together! Without an effective means to express ideas, concepts, concerns, instructions, share perceptions and questions, all other areas of non-technical behaviour are severely impacted.

How do we communicate? Without going into a lengthy theoretical discussion here, I've heard it said that around 7% of communication is verbal. The rest is made up of body language (55%) and tone and pitch (38%). Covering your body with scrubs and a mask doesn't exactly help either!

Have a think for a minute about how you communicate in the work environment.

How can you tell that your communication is effective? Other team members may have heard you, but have they understood the intent of the message?

How do you tell if your communications are not well received without the other person verbalizing it? What signs could you look for?

Do you look to see if they've received the message/instruction before going on to the next step?

What's your strategy if the message isn't understood the first time? Often, we simply raise the volume (I'm guilty of this on occasion) or slow our speech as if our colleagues suddenly have developed comprehension issues! It may simply require you to rephrase the statement.

All of the aircraft accidents mentioned in this book so far have, in varying degrees, pointed to breakdowns in communication as a contributing factor.

Air France 447, which had the instrument/airspeed malfunctions due to probe icing, had one pilot trying to make control inputs in an attempt to get the aircraft under control but did not *communicate* this action with the other pilot, leading to further confusion on the flight deck (this was exacerbated by the functionality of the Airbus' sidestick which, when one pilots moves it, it does not move the other pilot's sidestick control, unlike the traditional control column).

The massive disaster at Tenerife where two jumbo jets collided on the ground also highlighted communication issues as a causal factor, with English (the language used internationally in aviation) not being the native tongue of Air Traffic Control in the Canary Islands and the KLM flight crew. Non-standard phraseology in the initial airways clearance (using the phrase 'after takeoff' followed by heading and altitude instructions) lead the

KLM crew to believe they had been cleared for 'takeoff' when, in fact, they hadn't.

Even the VHF radios themselves potentially contributed to this accident in as much as no two parties could communicate concurrently, thus effectively blocking transmissions when two parties attempted to transmit at the same time.

As KLM started its takeoff roll and the First Officer transmitted that they were 'at takeoff' both the Pan AM flight crew and ATC reacted with their own transmissions in response the KLM, but neither were heard due to the limitations of the VHF radios.

The flight that crashed into Mt Erebus during an Antarctic scenic flight did not have crucial flight plan adjustments communicated to the flight crew. The crew were still under the impression that they were flying the old coordinates on the flight plan that they had been briefed on two weeks before the crash.

The DC-10 that crashed in Sioux following the complete loss of hydraulic power to the flight controls, greatly benefited from the high level of communication and teamwork between the flight crew themselves and with the aircraft and Air Traffic Control, saving many lives in the process.

The tenuous radio communication link used by Commander Jim Lovell and Director Gene Kranz was the only form of information sharing they had available, as they worked together to solve increasing complex and previously unknown problems resulting in their successful return of Apollo 13 to Earth.

Communication or the 'effective transfer of meaning' is a vital component of any safety related activity such as aviation or surgery.

Some situations are time critical, placing further pressure on messages to be verbalized and understood expeditiously. As pressure mounts, speech tends to become short and sharp as time is often critical. This can however, increase overall team workload as stress rises.

Do you change your normal delivery of information if under time pressure? If so, how, and is it effective?

Is it realistic for your team to simply know what you want and how you will react to changing scenarios?

Communication also has an enormous impact on the delivery and reception of training.

Sometimes, as an instructor, it's easy to feel frustrated when the trainee simply 'doesn't get it'!

It's also easy to put that responsibility of the training outcome onto the trainee.

In flight training, if a trainee pilot is having difficulty understanding a concept and/or reproducing a skill set, the responsibility rests firmly with the flight instructor who has to adapt to the needs and requirements of the trainee pilot.

Why isn't he/she getting this right? How should I change my delivery of information and/or style of training to allow the trainee to progress?

The 'how' will depend on the why!

The trainee might be under some psychological or physical stress or fatigue. They might have had a previous negative training outcome that is affecting their progress on this one. Or, they might just not 'get it' in the way it's being explained!

As we all perceive and learn in various ways, aural, visual, kinaesthetic or a combination of all of them, we, as instructors, may not be aware of the learning style of the trainee. It may take time to adjust to the learning styles of those under our guidance. I admit there are times when, despite our best efforts, trainees are, for whatever reason, unable to perform a task to a proficient standard.

I've often postponed a trainees' flight due to challenging weather conditions and had to complete the flight myself. Even in these situations, effective communication is crucial so that the trainee understood the context of my decision and not to take it as a negative judgement of his or her ability.

Of course, checking that information has in fact, been received and understood, is sometimes a challenge within itself. One technique I use is to ask the trainee to give me two new ideas or concepts that he/she will be taking away from todays' training. In most situations, the trainee will demonstrate their competence practically, but it doesn't hurt to ensure sound understanding exists.

Facilitation

One of the key aspects to any personal or professional development I've explored over the years, including my time as a flight instructor, is being aware of the power of asking good quality questions.

Adult learning principles decree that adults like to be involved in their own training, have previous experience that they like to use, and need to establish context and relevance to all learnings for them to be applied effectively.

Facilitation, or the ability of the facilitator to guide and encourage trainees to self-evaluate before giving constructive feedback as the instructor, ticks most of those adult learning boxes.

While actively encouraging trainees to self-assess, the instructor is also helping them learn to maintain effective situational awareness, of which self-awareness/assessment is a big part.

The main thing that sets facilitation apart from straight 'lecturing' is that facilitation is '*trainee* focused' NOT instructor focused.

The specific needs of the individual trainee can then be accounted for instead of labouring 'pet' subjects that the instructor feels comfortable teaching.

As mentioned previously, communication is the glue that holds all the other factors in place, the absence of which makes achievement of any level of competence or goals extremely unlikely.

The best tool, in my opinion, to 'grease the wheel' and ensure open, honest communication within your team, whilst maintaining a high level of effective situational awareness, is by asking timely, appropriate, targeted and relevant questions.

- With the given information before us, what options do we have?
- Which option do you feel more comfortable with?
- Have we forgotten anything here?
- Can we look at this another way?
- Where can we get more information?
- What could we have done differently?
- Why did that procedure go so well? So often we focus on areas that can be improved but sometimes reinforcing why things went well in a certain area can be extremely beneficial to the trainee.

The list of possible questions is endless, and the more you practice asking them, like any skill, the better you get at it! Just like any computer program, asking good quality questions usually results in getting good quality answers! Good stuff in, good stuff out.

If the answer doesn't come, maybe you need to ask a better question? I've experienced this sometimes during presentations while attempting to facilitate a discussion with a group but getting little in the way of feedback from the room. I take the responsibility for this lack of 'interaction' if you like, and once that responsibility is accepted, I can take steps to get a better outcome but asking better questions until I start to get a better, more interactive response.

Facilitation is a skill that takes a while to develop but is essential for effective training in any sphere of expertise.

I have also found, over many years of trying to ask good quality questions of my trainees, that I start to ask good quality questions of myself. My own personal self-assessment skills develop so that the habit of analysing alternatives and evaluating self-performance becomes natural.

Communication is the keystone for all the other aspects of human behaviour.

Part F – Threat and Error Management

On the flight deck, as we are briefing the crew for departure, an important part of that brief is to identify potential threats particular to that flight. I'm not talking about a 'security' type threat (hijack etc.) but rather any other key operational aspect that may have a detrimental effect on the flight on that day.

These threats could include adverse weather such as strong crosswinds, wet or icy runway, limited visibility, terrain close to the airport, or unserviceability's carried by the aircraft or airport facility such as lighting or navigation aid outages.

Back of the clock operations are another significant potential threat. Simply put, we are identifying potential threats from man, machine or environment.

But just identifying the threat is meaningless without mentioning mitigators i.e. how do we minimize the potential effect of these threats to the flight?

For example, if we identified that there was significant terrain around the airport, we might ensure one pilot has the 'terrain' function selected on his navigation display (this is a GPS backed terrain database which overlays onto our navigation screens effectively highlighting where the terrain is in relation to the departure flight path.)

We might also choose to maximize the climb angle of the aircraft until a safe altitude on departure, to get above the terrain as soon as possible.

We sometimes carry 'permissible unserviceability's' such as one thrust reverser inoperative (this is to allow the aircraft to get to an airport where repairs can be made.) There is a list of such unserviceability's' from each aircraft manufacturer that tells us what is allowed and what procedures we have to follow to operate without this equipment. Obviously, some equipment is necessary for every flight and therefore won't be on the list. In the case of an inoperative thrust reverser, we might talk about the effect that would have on runway length in the event of a return to this airfield or the handling characteristics in the case of a rejected takeoff (where the takeoff is aborted due to certain conditions such as engine failure or fire warnings.)

If the flight departs late at night, it might be prudent to identify that aspect alone as a potential threat to which appropriate mitigators might include maintaining a slow operational pace, strict adherence to standard operating procedures and reinforcing to the crew to speak up if any errors are detected.

Staying ahead of potential threats is key to a safe and effective operating environment.

The other side to the overall concept of threat and error management is minimizing errors. Hopefully by reviewing potential threats to the flight will in itself, greatly reduce the risk of making errors.

Errors, while rarely deliberate or wilful departures from standard procedures, are normally grouped into 'handling errors' (relating to flying, either manually or by using the aircrafts automatic systems, within the accepted flight tolerances), procedural errors or communication errors.

Strict adherence to standard operating procedures will greatly help, not only to minimize errors, but to aid in the detection and rectification of those errors.

For example, if the pilots had omitted to program the appropriate landing weight and flap setting into the flight management computer whilst performing their descent/ approach procedures, the descent checklist would detect this error and ensure compliance with procedures.

Plenty has been written on minimizing errors, but what about the ongoing effect of making those errors both procedurally and psychologically?

Some errors, if left undetected, may lead to others causing an 'error chain'. Forgetting to put the landing gear down until the automated 'gear not down' warning system is heard, may be a huge distraction to conducting a safe approach or go-around (especially if 'startle factor' occurs...).

As professional pilots, no-one likes to make errors, especially in front of other crew. Our pride is hurt and it can take a certain discipline to recover from those errors.

I've seen pilots make simple errors in a flight simulator exercise that normally would have little impact on the overall flight but have taken a huge emotional toll on the pilot as he or she comes to terms with their mistake.

This pilot may devote so much brain-space dwelling on that error, that it has a detrimental effect on the rest of the flight, often leading to further errors. One pilot making errors greatly increases the workload for the other pilot as they attempt to minimise the effect of the mistakes whilst being increasingly vigilant for others that may happen.

We do so much work on minimizing errors, but it's just as important to examine how we can recover from the errors we do make.

As a First Officer, I spent a lot of time in the flight simulator supporting pilots undergoing training for their Command. It was a great opportunity for me to see what worked and what didn't in terms of management style. I saw some pilots make simple errors but couldn't recover from the fact that they'd made them. It affected the rest of the exercise as they continued to think about their previous mistake.

I saw other pilots who also made errors, but had the ability and operational confidence to regroup, replan, and lead the operation to a successful outcome.

These pilots weren't *debilitated* by their mistakes. They appreciated the fact they we, as humans, are all capable of making errors. The key however, is to minimize the effect of those errors. Realizing that you have 'painted yourself into a corner' and are now focused on getting out.

Whether the error was caused by a lack of situational awareness, ineffective communication or a lack of perception of a given situation, there **must** be steps taken to break the error chain both procedurally and mentally to ensure a safe outcome overall.

A pilot who mishandles an approach becoming outside tolerances, realizes this and conducts a 'missed approach' or go-around should never be assessed negatively for these actions. As an instructor, I will always the reinforce to the trainees the merits of discontinuing an approach that becomes outside tolerance, regrouping and conducting a second stable approach and landing. The error has been recognized and the effect minimized.

Just having the confidence to admit that an error has been made is a great start to breaking the error chain!

As with all aspects of human factors, threat and error management is heavily reliant on effective communication, a workable authority gradient, effective leadership and teamwork. Each of these areas are inextricably linked and have an impact on the others.

- Can you identify potential threats to the operating theatre and your surgical team?

This list may include new technology being used for the first time, a recent change in team member which may alter the normal operating dynamic, fatigue after an already long surgical list, or the complexity of the procedure itself.

- What steps could you take to mitigate these threats?
- Would it be beneficial to consult with other team members to see if they can identify other potential threats?
- How do you minimise errors in the operating theatre?
- Once an error has been identified, how can you ensure that the mistake does not have a negative effect on the rest of the procedure?
- Do you think your team would be comfortable with verbalizing an error that you've made?
- How does making an error make you feel? This maybe a weird question but, in the safety of your own study, lounge room etc. you can be totally honest with yourself!

Even if you're not in the habit of making many errors, I feel it's really beneficial to examine the effect making an error can have on us. As I mentioned before, as professionals we pride ourselves in doing the absolute best job possible. We are also human beings and, as such, are subject to the effects of fatigue, outside influences such as domestic/financial problems etc. and these issues can find their way into our work space quite easily, making us more prone to errors. Maintaining a consistent threat and error management strategy is vital in recognizing potential issues that may have an effect on delivering the safest and best outcomes for those in our care.

3: DEALING WITH TECHNOLOGY

Rapid advances are being made in computerized technologies in almost every field of endeavour. MRI, fibre optics and laparoscopic techniques, robotics and prosthetics for the medical world and GPS navigation, autopilot technology, composite lightweight materials and weather forecasting in the aviation world.

But does advancing technology necessarily guarantee better and safer outcomes?

You'd like to think it does, but it comes with its own set of unique challenges…

For technology to be successfully implemented, three key aspects need to be covered effectively; training, understanding and support.

Part A – Training

Air France 447, Atlantic Ocean. June 1, 2009.

An Airbus A330 service from Rio de Janeiro in Brazil to Paris France in 2009, flight AF 447 entered an area of convective cloud and associated turbulence and icing at 33,000ft causing some important data gathering instruments (pitot tubes) to ice up and give erroneous information to the crew regarding airspeed and altitude.

The A330 is an 'envelope protected' aircraft which, simply put, in 'normal flight control law' protects itself from undesirable aircraft states such as stalling (disturbance of airflow over the wing resulting in a reduction in lift). The trouble starts however, when the data required for that envelope protection is corrupted in a situation like the icing of the pitot tubes experienced by AF 447.

Airspeed indications fluctuated wildly and warning sounds, including the stall warning, occurred. One of the flight crew attempted to respond to the inappropriately high airspeed indications by pulling the side stick control back (up) instead of forward (down) to correct the stall. Ergonomically, on the A330, when one pilot makes an input on the side stick, the other side stick does not move, unlike the conventional control yoke where both control columns move irrespective of which pilot puts the control input in, making it difficult for pilots to monitor each other's inputs (especially in the dark).

The Captain, who was in the crew rest station at the time, made it back to the flight deck and attempted to regain control of the now fully stalled and rapidly plummeting A330. Unfortunately, this was not successful and the aircraft crashed into the ocean killing all 228 passengers and crew on board.

Final reports into the accident indicated the flight crew on duty that night lacked the practical training in high altitude aircraft handling and an understanding of the aerodynamic characteristics approaching the stall, to successfully recover from this situation.

This lack of understanding may have stemmed from an over reliance on the 'envelope protections' of the A330, thus potentially overshadowing the need for training in the skills required to deal with high altitude events such as this one.

Since AF447, high altitude and stall recovery, combined with unreliable airspeed training has been greatly enhanced by airline operators around the world.

Flight simulators can now be used to provide this training safely. They are capable of reproducing a variety of instrument and navigational malfunctions similar to the conditions experienced by Air France 447 allowing pilots to recognize these situations and practice the required recovery manoeuvres.

Flight simulators are equipped with the latest visual graphics, sound effects and programming to allow training in dealing with almost every potential malfunction on the aircraft.

Simulator lesson plans include not just the technical side of aircraft handling and automation management, but also creating real time flight scenarios where crew can experience and practice their 'non-technical' skills (often referred to as Crew Resource Management or CRM). Medical simulation devices are already in use for training purposes in a number of areas such as advanced life support and resuscitation.

One simply cannot hope to safely operate any piece of technology without the required skill set. This skill set must include not only the ability to effectively operate new equipment, but also must ensure the user is fully aware of the limitations, potential traps and characteristics that could lead to the equipment delivering a less than optimum outcome. New equipment training often assumes that the user has prior base line knowledge of previously utilized procedural techniques, so that they can revert to those techniques if use of the new technologies goes astray.

Pilots are regularly assessed in the flight simulator and the aircraft to ensure knowledge and flight skills are kept up to date and proficiency standards maintained.

Four times per year, airline pilots have to successfully complete simulator training and testing to both reinforce previously acquired skills and, through "evidence-based training", train in situations that may have recently occurred in airline operations globally. (imagine having to sit your driving test every three months!)

Once per year, most airlines also check the proficiency of pilots in the real aircraft, with the Training Captain sitting in the back seat observing and assessing actual line operations and standards.

Now this level of scrutiny is obviously impractical in the medical/surgical professions, however the concept of the regular examination of current standards by training personnel is key to ensuing that those standards are maintained across any area of expertise.

- Have you ever trained another doctor in the use of a piece of equipment e.g. a laparoscopic instrument? Did you certify them as 'proficient' at the end of the training?
- What ongoing liability might you have for that trainees' future use of that equipment?
- Are you aware if that practitioner kept up with manufacturers updates, refreshers etc.?
- Once you deem someone competent, how far does your responsibility extend in the future usage of that equipment?
- How can you ensure that the trainee will maintain the level of proficiency that was demonstrated in your presence?

Training in the use of any new equipment and/or technologies is critical.

Part B – Understanding new systems

'*Understanding*' is the next level in any education piece, for it is simply not enough to be able to 'press the right buttons' to operate equipment effectively, especially when things don't go to plan. Initial training will normally only allow you to perform basic functions of the technologies only. Without an underlying appreciation of 'how' systems work and respond to various scenarios, one does not possess the skills to confidently use the device in a range of complicated situations. One needs to fully appreciate not only the 'pure science' behind the new technology but also the 'applied science' which puts practical context to the everyday use of the equipment. From an instructors' point of view, we call this 'value adding', or showing how to apply theoretical principles to actual practice.

As mentioned above, a lack of *understanding* of the situation regarding unreliable speed and stall recognition was named as a causal factor in Air France 447. Initial training alone may not be enough to ensure effective *understanding* both at the time of initial training and the ongoing knowledge maintenance required to keep up with advancing technologies.

There were two separate but similar aircraft accidents involving the Airbus A300 in 1994 and 1998 respectively where, on final approach, the 'Takeoff-Go around' switch was accidentally pressed. This action results in a large increase in engine thrust to normally allow the pilot to conduct the 'missed approach' or go-around manoeuvre. This manoeuvre is done when a pilot decides to 'abort' the landing attempt and come around for another try. There could be various reasons for this 'abort', adverse weather conditions at the airfield, aircraft on the runway etc.

In these cases, however, the pilots attempted to manually override the Take-off Go-around automated function, with the downward pressure on the control column resulting in the autopilot 'trimming' this force with *opposite* direction nose 'up' trim. Unfortunately, the human interface was acting against the automation and when the autopilot finally disconnected, the aircraft pitched up violently until it stalled and crashed.

There appeared to be a lack of *understanding* of the automated systems; systems that were doing exactly what they were supposed to be doing.

Whilst I'm sure this manoeuvre would have been *trained* in the flight simulator as the pilots were learning about this new aircraft, simply practicing a trained manoeuvre doesn't necessarily mean that a full appreciation or *understanding* of the technology exists.

Flight instructors are assessed regularly in their delivery of training both in the simulator and the aircraft, again to ensure that standards are maintained. Trainers are encouraged to 'value add' during all the various flight sequences at every opportunity, with the hope of increasing pilots *understanding* of the technology and principles. Often this 'extra' insight is based on the instructors' experience and the benefit of seeing many crews operate flight sequences in the simulator. This additional training input should be ongoing in a pilots' career, so that the initial training is enhanced by an increased level of understanding and application of systems and concepts.

Pilots have access to the 'pure science' in their flight manuals and other reference material. They then learn the 'applied science' by benefiting from the experience and 'value adding' from the instructors.

Technology has the potential to become a hindrance and produce less than desirable outcomes if that theoretical AND practical applications of the equipment are not fully understood.

Part C – Support services

I don't think there's ever been a time when I haven't had to 'consult the manual' be it the Aircraft Flight Manual when dealing with issues on the flight deck, or the DVD recording manual for how to record a TV show! (that's what kids are for right?)

Initial training simply isn't enough to cover all of the possible scenarios and features available of any device, so ongoing support services are vital to the successful implementation of new technologies, particularly if it involves software updating (which often changes regularly).

These support services are vital to ensure the operators of these technologies are aware of the constantly changing enhancements and experiences of other operators, particularly if the technology is very new.

Mt Erebus, Antarctica. November 28, 1979.

On the 28th of Nov 1979, flight TE901, an Air New Zealand DC-10 aircraft departed on a sightseeing flight to Antarctica.

The pilots had attended a flight briefing some 19 days before the journey, a briefing which included an audio-visual presentation of the expected flight path. This path had been flown many times and provided the public with a close-up view of the Antarctic landscape.

Unfortunately, the night before the departure of flight TE901, Air New Zealand's flight planning staff altered one of the flight plan computer 'waypoints' (a programmed navigation mark that is inserted into the aircrafts' flight management computer) in an attempt to fix a small error that had been discovered. The intended fix was to alter the aircrafts flight path by 2 nautical miles (just under 4 kilometres). Instead however, the effect of the change by the flight planning staff actually resulted in a flight path deviation of nearly 30 nautical miles (over 50kms)! The pilots were unaware that this change had been made and still held the 'mental model' of the flight they were expecting from the pre- flight briefing. Topographical maps were not given to the pilots on the day of the flight.

Previous crews had actually been using the original plan containing the error but had been blessed with clear skies on the day of their flights, enabling them to be aware of the high terrain in the area.

Sadly though, flight TE901 did not have such luck with the conditions that day, where extensive cloud cover made them totally reliant on the computer flight plan, a plan which had been altered the night before.

The pilots flew the programmed track, and upon reaching the point where it was designated safe to descend to achieve the desired scenic views of Antarctica, descended with an expectation that the weather would clear and for them to be positioned over McMurdo Sound and clear of terrain. Instead, the aircraft flew directly into Mount Erebus, an active volcano, killing all 257 passengers and crew on board.

So, even though the pilots had been *trained* in the operation of the navigation systems of their DC10 aircraft, and they *understood* the technology behind the systems, circumstances beyond that training and understanding occurred external to their sphere of influence, i.e. the flight planning support services , had provided inaccurate data for the computer flight plan, resulting in this being the 'dominant' causal factor leading the accident (ref; Justice McMahon in his report in the 1980 Royal Commission into the event).

Support services need to be reliable, available and able to provide the absolute latest technological updates, to consistently allow the operator to achieve and maintain proficiency in the use of the new equipment.

Without *training*, *understanding* and *support services* firmly and effectively in place and *ongoing*, there is potential for technology to produce less than desirable outcomes.

Ask yourself, has there ever been a time when you have used a piece of new equipment/technology and you wished you could have had more training, to enhance your understanding of the tool or system, or even needed greater support from the supplier/manufacturer? It doesn't need to be in a professional capacity to come up with examples of these potential shortfalls! Think back to the complex TV recording devices on the market or programming your smartphone.

I guess the biggest takeaway from this chapter is simply to ask yourself, when presented with an opportunity to utilize new technology of any kind…

Have I had sufficient *training* to safely and effectively use it?

Do I fully *understand* the capabilities and potential shortcomings etc. of the equipment?

Can I rely on the *ongoing support* of the manufacturer to ensure it is being used with the most up to date information possible?

This overwhelming surge of technological advancement doesn't come without its challenges. Incorporating new equipment into your practice comes with a commitment to utilise that new technology to its maximum capability whilst still ensuring safety for those in your care.

4: USE OF CHECKLISTS

This subject often comes up in my presentations to groups of surgeons and much has already been written on this aspect of practice.

In any field of endeavor, as ever-increasing volumes of subject theory and practical application of knowledge are derived, so too does the burden placed upon professionals in those fields to assimilate this knowledge into daily practice. Put simply, our world has become more complicated!

Checklists can provide a structure for, not only the routine procedures, but also in the management of complex scenarios. In aviation, 'Non-normal' checklists (which aircrew refer to for various system failures) clarify the management of the scenario by not only outlining particular procedural steps, but also highlighting the ramifications of that failed system on other aircraft systems as well.

For example, a failure of the wing flaps (responsible for changing the shape or camber of the wing to allow for low speed flight phases such as takeoff and landing) to deploy, may have an effect on the autopilots' ability to make an automatic landing in low visibility conditions such as fog. The checklist will highlight this ramification which will influence the crews' decision on the choice of airports available for landing.

As aircraft systems become more complicated, aircrew rely more heavily on using checklists to manage non-normal events.

The pre-flight sequence alone consists of hundreds of procedural steps, calculations, switching etc. A checklist is read immediately prior to engine start, taxiing the aircraft to the takeoff position and indeed the takeoff itself. These checklists usually consist of a few important items that have a direct impact on the safe continuance of the flight.

Other phases of flight, descent, approach and landing also, after various procedural steps have been completed, have their own checklist to confirm that crucial items have been completed.

Does the use of checklists provide a 100% guaranteed safety net to catch all errors? No, it doesn't, but certainly goes a long way to minimise errors especially when conditions such as fatigue, complacency (repetitive environment) distraction etc. exist.

Errors still occur even when utilizing checklists. These errors include doing the checklist from memory, doing the wrong checklist, doing the right checklist incorrectly, or simply not completing a checklist.

Other time critical checklists dealing with non-normal events such as engine fire have memory checklists to be conducted as soon as the flight path is under control. These checklists are usually fairly short and involve taking immediate steps to minimise the effect of the failure condition.

Equally important though, memory checklists items assist in dealing with 'startle effect', commonly referred to as the fight or flight physiological effect on the human body in response to an unexpected event. Heart rate, blood sugar, cortisol and respiratory rates all skyrocket to prepare the body for confrontation all at the expense of cognitive thought which goes on the back burner for around 30-45 seconds!

Having a rehearsed memory checklist, one that is practiced regularly in the flight simulator, tends to cut through that cognitive 'blackout', carrying out initial steps to put the aircraft in a safe configuration until further trouble shooting can be done.

Now I have, while presenting to surgical teams in the past, sensed a reluctance to utilize checklists, almost as if it demeans the surgeons' ability and/or prowess and could be interpreted as a 'crutch' or memory aid.

The key here, I feel, is Gawande's statement on complexity. When I flew my little Cessna 150 single engine aircraft around the training area in Taree when I was learning to fly, there were still checklists to complete, but they were very short and simple ones compared to the operation of the wide-bodied international jet aircraft capable of carrying hundreds of passengers greater distances at much higher altitudes. As complexity increases, so does the importance of reference and memory checklists to safely and effectively operate these systems.

Checklists provide punctuation marks in a procedure where the overall situation and progress can be assessed, a chance to 'refocus' if you like, on the task at hand. This positive control of the 'tempo' of a situation is vital to ensure that the situation itself doesn't dictate your operational pace. I've seen many situations in the flight simulator where pilots are put under pressure by various non-normal scenarios causing them to rush techniques to quickly resolve the problem. This is because the event itself is governing the pace, NOT the pilots. This "tail wagging the dog' phenomenon must be countered somehow to allow procedures, trouble shooting and flying techniques to be completed correctly and appropriately.

Having a standard checklist whereby one pilot verbalizes an item and expects a standard response from the other pilot, also provides a degree of cover to guard against subtle incapacitation. If the responses to a checklist vary from the standard expected, pilots are trained to question the possible causes of the variation to mitigate a simple procedural error or to flag a pilot experiencing some form of incapacitation. (e.g. minor stroke, diabetic event etc.) It also puts them 'on guard' to monitor possible non-standard behaviour in the other crew member, which thankfully, is very rare indeed!

There will always be the potential for a situation that goes beyond the scope of any checklist and requires the skills, experience and knowledge of the operator to deal with it. Point in case was the Qantas flight QF32 Airbus A380 which had the uncontained engine failure that caused multiple failure messages to be generated, the sum of which created a situation outside of the normal scope of the checklists. Management of this critical scenario included thinking beyond each individual checklist as, similar to the case of Apollo 13, this particular scenario had not been envisaged or trained for. Each checklist dealt with specific system failures. There was not a checklist for the combined ramifications of the external damage caused by the engine failure.

Checklists are a very useful 'tool' and that's *all* they are, a 'tool', not something designed to restrict creativity or expression, but merely to ensure the 'big ticket' items are covered and standard operating procedures are adhered to.

As an airline Captain, dealing with increasingly complex systems and ever advancing technologies, I rely on checklist information to enhance my overall operational management and capability. They are very useful tools to diagnose non-normal aircraft systems events, guiding pilots through the appropriate procedural steps and stages without adversely affecting other systems in the process, and to configure the aircraft for approach and landing.

Checklists also ensure that, within normal parameters, pilots are following Standard Operating Procedures or SOPs, making it relatively seamless when operating with different crews every trip.

Checklists form the backbone of our operational management structure, a structure which, if attempted from memory alone, would potentially struggle in these complex, arduous and rapidly changing times.

5: QUICK REFERENCE CHECKLISTS

On most flight decks, although with the trend away from paper manuals, these are getting rarer, we have what's known as 'Quick Reference Checklists' which contain important time critical checklists, performance information, required equipment lists and safety announcements to the cabin. It doesn't contain all our technical information, just the things we might need in a hurry!

This chapter is your own set of 'Quick Reference Checklists'

(and I really hope you do reference these questions regularly...)

I have included a summary of all the questions I've put to you in this book.

The answers will very much depend on your type of work, team dynamic, personality etc. but as I've already stated, any form of development requires asking good quality questions!

As the name suggests, these are quick reference checklists in a format to make it easy to focus on a particular area.

I encourage you to refer to these checklists as you examine your own working environment.

Authority Gradient Checklist

1. What's the angle of the authority gradient in your workplace environment?
2. Do your team members feel comfortable expressing concerns and giving constructive input?
3. Have you ever discussed strategies to combat the possibility of subtle incapacitation with your team members?
4. Is it possible that some members of surgical teams might not be willing to give input, for a variety of reasons, when things aren't going so well?

Situational Awareness (SA) Checklist

1. Who is responsible for maintaining SA in the operating theatre environment? **(who has the big picture?)**
2. How is the perception of new data affecting the procedure shared with all team members to ensure the big picture is a common vision? **(also referred to as the 'shared mental model')**
3. How are changes to the individual situations communicated to the rest of the team, anaesthetic staff, life support techs, nursing staff etc. to ensure everyone is on the same page?
4. What factors could impede maintaining good SA? **(hint: fatigue, unexpected technical complexity, less than optimum authority gradient)**

5.   How do we regain SA once it's been lost? **(Clear communication. Get back to basics, seek information, rebuild the platform, reassess, replan, find some 'clear air'...)**

Decision Making Checklist

1.   How are decisions made in your operating theatre or medical practice?
2.   How do you review the effectiveness/appropriateness of those decisions?
3.   How are those decisions communicated with the rest of the team members?
4.   Do you feel that you need to justify your decisions?
5.   Would your team members express anything that wasn't clear and/or concerns about any decisions made?
6.   How would you handle it if they did express concern?

Leadership Checklist

1.   What is your leadership style?
2.   How effective do you think it is?
3.   How would you know if it was breaking down?
4.   Do you see yourself as the head of the team or as 'the leader'?
5.   Does your team see you as a leader?

Teamwork Checklist

1.   How effectively does your team function?
2.   If they function really well, why?
3.   What makes them a great team?

4. If you could think of one thing that would enhance teamwork in your workplace, what would it be?
5. How does your team rate its effectiveness and why?

Communication Checklist

1. How can you tell that your communication style is effective?
2. How do you tell if your communications are not well received without the other person verbalizing it?
3. Do you look to see if team members have received the message/instruction before going on to the next step?
4. What's your strategy if messages or instructions aren't clearly understood the first time?
5. Does your communication style change if pressure increases?
6. When training others, are you an instructor or a facilitator?

Threat and Error Management Checklist

1. Can you identify potential threats in the operating theatre and to your surgical team and patients?
2. What steps could you take to mitigate these threats?
3. Would it be beneficial to consult with other team members to see if they can identify other potential threats?
4. How do you minimize errors in the operating theatre?
5. When are errors most likely to occur?

6. Once an error has been identified, how can you ensure that the error does not have a negative ongoing effect on the rest of the procedure?
7. Do you think your team would be comfortable with verbalizing an error that you've made?
8. How does making an error make you feel?

Technology Checklist

1. Does advancing technology necessarily guarantee better and safer outcomes?
2. Have I had **adequate training** to safely and effectively use new equipment?
3. Do I fully **understand** the capabilities, potential shortcomings etc. of new technology?
4. Can I rely on the **ongoing support** from the manufacturer to ensure the equipment is being used with the most up to date information possible?
5. How do I ensure that these new skills and competencies are maintained with existing team members and how do we train new team members in new technologies?

CONCLUSION

One final story.

A few years ago, I was departing Hong Kong for Perth in a fully laden Boeing 767. The First Officer was the pilot flying and, when he attempted to retract the flaps after take-off, we received a warning message from the aircrafts' EICAS (engine indicating and crew alerting system), informing us that the leading-edge slats (part of the movable wing flap system that allows for greater lift during takeoff and slower approach speeds during landing) were stuck partially extended on one side of the wing. The larger trailing edge flaps had retracted normally but a portion of leading-edge slats were still extended on one wing. This is known as a slat asymmetry. In itself, not a huge safety concern, as an electric back up to the normal hydraulic system was available to retract the slats.

We informed Air Traffic Control that we would like to level off to run some checklists and troubleshoot our problem. I was expecting the electric back up to retract the slats and we could continue to Perth. Continuing to Perth with the slats still extended was not allowed as it would require both high speed and high altitude flight, not possible with wing slats extended.

Unfortunately, checklist action was not successful in retracting the slats leading us into a return to land scenario back in Hong Kong.

Before this could happen however, there was much to be done: ATC had to be notified of our intentions, fuel had to be jettisoned as we were well above the maximum landing weight (this also has to be coordinated with ATC to ensure the aircraft is within the prescribed fuel dumping area), cabin crew and passengers had to be updated and the company notified to arrange ground handling. My flight crew team were busy organising these various tasks whilst, at all times, ensuring someone was focusing on flying the aircraft!

I briefed the cabin crew to expect a normal, although slightly faster approach and landing (more on this later) and they went about their tasks preparing the cabin and reassuring the passengers.

After the fuel jettison and weight reduction was completed, we set about the task of preparing for the approach. With this particular issue, where we had little in the way of leading-edge slats available, we were expecting a slightly faster approach speed to compensate for this anomaly. This was on the assumption that we still had the large training edge wing flaps available to allow for slower approach speeds for landing.

What happened next however, was not expected. As we attempted to extend the trailing edge flaps, we discovered that these too were stuck using both the hydraulic AND electric backup systems! Now this complicated matters and required further thought. We informed Air Traffic Control that we'd like to remain in the holding pattern until further advised until we processed the implications of our predicament. Simply put, the aircraft had no functioning leading or trailing edge devices to slow the aircraft down to the normal approach speed. Everything else on the aircraft was working perfectly such as engines etc. and the weather was crystal clear in the Hong Kong area with very little wind.

Interestingly enough, around six months previously, I had, along with a colleague of mine, written an article specifically dealing with a range of flap and slat malfunctions, including no flaps/slats at all. This was an incredible coincidence bearing in mind the situation in which I was now faced. To research this paper, we had flown some 8 hours in the flight simulator, experiencing first-hand the characteristics of each malfunction. Whilst, in my regular job as a trainer in the flight simulator, I was reasonably familiar with these sequences, it was invaluable to have had such recent practice under my belt!

While we were in the holding pattern, I gave regular updates to the passengers and cabin crew to reassure them that we were dealing with this situation and that the aircraft was in a safe configuration.

So, with all the appropriate checklists completed, we started examining how we were going to fly the approach. Checklists, while a great tool, are limited in that they give you information on systems status, switch positions, approach speeds etc. mainly dealing with the 'what' but give you little guidance in the 'how'.

'How' we were going to fly the approach and landing, took further input.

Simply put, we had to fly the approach around 45 knots (nautical miles per hour), or 83 kilometres per hour faster than the normal approach speed.

At this faster speed, there was a lot to consider as rate of descent, landing and stopping technique all had to be modified for the faster speed.

We, myself and my two first officers on board that night, explored as many options and permutations of this problem as we could think of including, how to assess rate of closure close to the ground at high speed, the effect of 'ground rush' as we had already been airborne and dealing with this problem for some hours and it was 3am local time, being able to bring the aircraft to a stop with the runway length available and without overheating the brakes.

With the combined experience we had on board that night, we came up with a plan, informed Air Traffic Control that we were ready for the approach, did a final check that we were all fully prepared for the task at hand, and commenced the approach.

The almost flapless aircraft at its final approach speed of around 185kts, handled exactly as it had done in the simulator. The pilot monitoring verbalised the altitude indications from around 300ft to the ground (the aircraft automatically calls "100.......50......30......." but he did it earlier to help gauge rate of closure).

We used all the available runway after landing and taxied into our gate.

After further liaison with ground staff, engineering, cabin crew, passengers etc. we made our way to the hotel. On the way however, we conducted our own debrief; a long hard look at how things went.

I was really interested in hearing how the other flight crew found the event and was pleased to hear that they didn't feel rushed at any stage, communications were clear and included all relevant parties and that they felt comfortable giving input and suggestions during the event. We gathered as much information was we could to aid the troubleshooting process (ATC, Engineering, checklists and aircraft manuals) formulated a plan, but, most importantly, we always had a plan 'B', reinforcing regularly, that if any of us thought plan 'A' was going pear shaped, to speak up, we can discontinue the approach and start over.

During the approach planning numerous threats were identified (high approach speed, the possible effect of 'ground rush' visual illusions in the landing phase, fatigue to name a few) and mitigators identified to deal with each one.

We made certain someone was always focused on flying the aircraft and that we regularly summarised the present situation to ensure that the 'big picture' was maintained and communicated to everyone including those in the cabin.

The authority gradient was such that all crew members felt comfortable to raise concerns and give input.

Our teamwork ensured that everyone had important jobs, not the least being monitoring each other. The cabin crew team ensured that the passengers were reassured and fully briefed. They had revised their emergency drills and were ready to swing into action of required. Thankfully, it wasn't.

Decisions were made only after careful consideration of all factors and ramifications associated with our problem.

The successful return to land in Hong Kong that night made me extremely proud of my team and was a great reminder of the significance, relevance and effectiveness of the Human Factors training we had received in various forms over the years.

As a final take 'takeaway' to sum up the key points, I'd like to offer the following 6 steps to enhance what you already do...

1) Be open to the idea of change.
2) Establish an *effective* 'authority gradient'. Be aware that this gradient may be compromised if multiple specialities are involved in the procedure.

3) Have an incapacitation plan. Discuss with your team exactly how to react and communicate if they think something's not right.

4) Utilise the benefits of checklists.

5) Encourage feedback. Maybe a quick informal debrief after each case of what went well and what could have been done differently?

6) Make human factors a *priority*. Simply being aware and vigilant of potential threats and considerations that each day may bring will enhance the effectiveness of 'human factors' in your operating environment.

It is my great hope that somewhere in the preceding pages you've read something that resonated for you; whether it's simply reinforcing things you do well already, refreshing some information that you've already heard but needed reviewing, or concepts, as a leader in a surgical/medical practice that you hadn't considered before.

The Human Factors principles explored in this book are universally relevant anytime and anywhere human beings are involved in any activity. They can equally be applied to sporting groups, corporate teams or wherever people work together to achieve a common goal.

I can honestly say that the study of Human Factors and behaviour gets more interesting, challenging and inspiring the longer I'm involved with it. It not only enhances our ability to train pilots effectively in many different scenarios, but its' overall applicability to all aspects of our lives, both professional and personal makes it extremely worthwhile.

Enjoy exploring 'why we do what we do'. The benefits are well worth it.

Thank you again for investing your time and effort.

I really look forward to any feedback you may have.

Cheers…

Geoff Hay

REFERENCES

Ketchikan, Alaska NTSB report AAR-76-24

Tenerife report by the Subsecretaria De Aviacion Civil, Spain

Cali, report DCA96RA020

Portland, NTSB report AAR-79-7

Hudson River NTSB report AAR-10/03

Sioux City NTSB report AAR-90-06

Air France 447- Bureau d'Entquetes Et d'Analyses

Justice McMahon Final Report Royal Commission Mt Erebus disaster 1980.

ACKNOWLEDGEMENT

I would like to thank Dr Philip Hayes, Dr Adam Mahoney and Dr Bernard Kelly for their expert technical help, support and feedback in producing this book.